BROOKLYN ZOO

Doubleday

NEW YORK   LONDON   TORONTO   SYDNEY   AUCKLAND

ZOO
BROOKLYN

The Education of a Psychotherapist

DARCY LOCKMAN

Grateful acknowledgment is made to the following for permission to reprint
previously published material:

Alfred Publishing Co., Inc.: Excerpt from "Brooklyn Zoo" by Ol' Dirty
Bastard and Derrick Harris, copyright © 1995 by Warner-Tamerlane
Publishing Corp. (BMI), Wu-Tang Publishing (BMI), and Bright Summit
Music (ASCAP). All rights on behalf of itself and Wu-Tang Publishing
administered by Warner-Tamerlane Publishing Corp. All rights reserved.
Reprinted by permission of Alfred Publishing Co., Inc.

NYP Holdings, Inc.: Excerpt from "B'klyn Psych Ward a Horror Show:
Suit" by Stefanie Cohen (*New York Post*, May 4, 2007). Reprinted by
permission of NYP Holdings, Inc.

Book design by Maria Carella
Jacket design by Emily Mahon
Jacket photograph © Tamara Staples

Library of Congress Cataloging-in-Publication Data
Lockman, Darcy, 1972–
Brooklyn zoo : the education of a psychotherapist / Darcy Lockman.—
1st ed.
p. cm.
1. Lockman, Darcy, 1972– 2. Psychotherapists—United States—
Biography. 3. Psychotherapists—In-service training. I. Title.
RC438.6.L63A3 2012
616.89'14092—dc23
[B]   2011043755

ISBN 978-0-385-53428-4

MANUFACTURED IN THE UNITED STATES OF AMERICA

1   3   5   7   9   10   8   6   4   2

First Edition

For George and Liv

I'm the one-man army, Ason
I never been tookin' out, I keep MCs lookin' out
I drop science like Cosby droppin' babies
Enough to make a nigga go crazy
In the G Building, takin' all types of medicines
Your ass thought you were better than
Ason, I keep planets in orbit
While I be comin' with deeper and more shit
Enough to make ya, break ya, shake ya ass.

—*"Brooklyn Zoo," by onetime Kings County Hospital psych patient Ol' Dirty Bastard*

A few months before I began the yearlong clinical internship necessary to complete my doctorate in psychology, my sister, a voracious reader, suggested I write this book. I went into psychology after some years spent as a magazine writer with the vague notion that I would eventually write about my field for a popular audience, so when she made her suggestion, I thought it was a good idea, and then I was never without my notebook during my time at Kings County Hospital. While names and identifying information of the people in this book have been changed, most of what is recounted here comes directly from my careful and copious notes.

BROOKLYN ZOO

PROLOGUE: THE G BUILDING

IT WAS THE MIDDLE OF A JUNE SO HOT YOU WOULDN'T WISH it on anyone, the last weeks of the last month of my internship year at Kings County Hospital. I was in a gypsy cab—the only kind of hired car to be found on the streets of East Flatbush— on my way to a job interview at a clinic in another marginalized Brooklyn neighborhood. ("The worst neighborhood you'll ever work in," the psychologist doing the hiring told me over the phone.) It was late in the afternoon when I flagged the driver down outside the hospital. Looking at the Kings County ID hanging low around my neck, he asked me where specifically I worked.

"G Building," I said, waiting for some version of what I knew by then would follow.

"Oh." He made eye contact, then looked away. "You work with the cuckoos."

I was pleased to be able to discern the driver's nationality, Haitian, from his intonation. Almost a year of working in that West Indian neighborhood had taught me to greet others with a smile and slow "good morning," and to distinguish the Jamaican lilt from the St. Lucian, the Haitian drawl from the Guyanese. I was less pleased with his words. After almost a year of working in and around the hospital's inpatient adult psychiatric building—known locally as G—I took them personally.

"They're just like everyone else," I said. He didn't reply. I protested further: "We all have our problems."

I would not convince him. Seven years of graduate school and just a dissertation short of doctor, I was only myself beginning to understand the elusive continuum that runs from psychosis to neurosis, from the wildly manic to the mildly depressive. The driver's attitude toward the mentally ill—the cuckoos—pervaded the neighborhood, if not the borough, the city, the country. We disdain in others what we disavow in ourselves.

From the beginning of my internship at Kings County Hospital, that much hadn't been hard to get. I had been a psychology intern for less than a week when I first learned the lore of the G Building from a Caribbean X-ray technician who was herself just starting at Kings County Hospital. We were at new-employee orientation, waiting together for an elevator. She was friendly. Everyone in East Flatbush was so friendly. After more than a decade spent in New York City neighborhoods where even a wan smile and a nod toward a neighbor recognized on the street were taken as intrusions, I had to make a conscious switch into that brand of solicitude. For me it was like the initial movement of a tape deck right as you pushed play. It felt effortful.

"You're a psychologist?" the X-ray tech asked, reading from my ID, which actually said "psychologist-in-training," but that was a mouthful. When I told her yes, she asked where in the hospital I would be working. Each of the buildings on the square mile of Kings County's campus was lettered, in no order that I could make out. J next to N. T next to A. "G Building," I told her. She laughed. I waited. When she stopped, she asked, not unkindly: "That's a real place?"

I looked puzzled, and she continued. "I grew up around here," she explained. " 'G Building' was like this slang. Instead of saying someone was crazy, you might say, 'He belongs in G Building.' Or some kids, if they were acting up, their parents might say, 'If you don't behave, we're going to send you to G Building.' I'd always heard that. I just didn't know G Building actually existed."

I was there to tell her that it did.

CHAPTER ONE

MY RELATIONSHIP WITH PSYCHOLOGY BEGAN WHEN I WAS eight. My mother started seeing a therapist she called Sylvia, and soon enough my father began going, too, after—as he would tell me many years later—my mom suggested the problems he was having in their marriage were not solely about her. What my mother meant was that my father was reexperiencing old feelings from his earliest formative relationship in the context of a new and different one. In other words, he felt treated by his wife how he'd felt treated by his mother. No one who knew my grandmother Mina (who openly derided every gift she'd ever gotten and had once shown up at my parents' apartment with just-purchased underwear for her newly wed son) could have imagined my father's old feelings to be benevolent. So my parents embarked on separate journeys of self-understanding, which I inferred allowed them to remain together. It was 1981, and we lived in the western suburbs of Detroit. Ronald Reagan had just become the country's first divorced president, and many of the fathers on our street were moving on. That therapy had facilitated my family's escape from the hovering menace of dissolution was no small thing to me.

And so I became curious about psychotherapy, but I never asked my parents to describe it. Like all of the adult concerns that evoked pointed interest in me, it seemed illicit. I also wanted badly to discourage all open discussion of their latest pastime, lest they feel comfortable enough to mention it in front of my friends, whose families I vehemently believed had stepped straight off the soundstages of the late-1950s sitcoms I'd seen in reruns. That my parents went to therapy became one more dreary secret that I added to a list, though what I was really most desperate to keep under wraps was how much they disliked me. Were others to know, they could only reject me as well.

Not long after they started seeing Sylvia, my mother went back to school to become a social worker, a therapist herself. I was in the fourth grade and my sister in kindergarten, and though my mom had once been a teacher, she'd been at home, more or less, since I was born. After her graduation from social work school, she started seeing patients, and like anyone else she would talk about her work. Her stories were more anecdotes than case presentations, but I didn't know enough to distinguish between the two. By the time I got to college, I assumed psych classes could only be superfluous, and I refused to sign up for any, defying all expectations of my gender and ethnicity. But also, as determined as I was at eighteen and twenty and even twenty-five to be sublimely unlike my mother, it never crossed my mind that I would become a therapist. I thought I'd be a lawyer—like my father.

It did occur to me to become a patient. The first time was my senior year of college after my mom suggested it. She thought I was "too anxious," a pronouncement I felt she might have delivered in any number of gentler ways, but still I considered it. She had colleagues near my campus in Ann Arbor, and she gave me a number. I called and got an answering machine but could not think of a thing to say. The second time was a couple of years later. I had finished undergrad and moved to New York to take an internship at a rock-and-roll magazine, but more to the point to live somewhere exciting. If things were going fine on paper, I often felt rotten. I couldn't make any sense of myself. One lesson I had learned from half-listened-to conversations from my adolescence was that there were a lot of bad therapists out there, and so I got another referral, from a friend of my mother's who knew a psychologist in Manhattan. I made an appointment but showed up on the wrong day, leaving Dr. Aronoff's office in angry tears when nobody answered the buzzer. As I walked south on Fifth Avenue along the park on the way back to the entertainment magazine where I had by then become an editorial assistant, I thought, "I am trying so hard and still cannot get any help," a masochist's mantra.

Years later I would learn from the therapist's side of the experience that the way in which a patient begins the therapy relationship is a proclamation of sorts—a snapshot of what he or she is struggling with—and I sometimes thought back on the way I began my own treatment. When I called Dr. Aronoff after that first afternoon to tell her that I'd traveled all the way from midtown at her behest just to find her absent, I was demonstrating this expectation: I would be the victim here and she my giddy torturer. "I teach on that day," I remember her responding kindly. "I don't think I would have scheduled an appointment then." Look now, she was alerting me, we have some other options.

What relieved me most in those first years with Dr. Aronoff was a nascent appreciation for my own internal consistency. Where my feelings had once seemed arbitrary and free-floating as particles of dust, it was now clear that they related to one another and also to the entire span of my backstory. As I had grown up fed and clothed and never so much as smacked on the bottom, it was easy to maintain a dogged belief that everything had been fine. It hadn't felt fine, but I'd learned to ignore that—hands over my ears as I hummed—because certainly that was my fault, a confirmation of my innate and immutable decrepitude. Only slowly and with Dr. Aronoff's listening could I begin to know more about my old feelings and the imprint those feelings had left.

I'd been lucky enough to stumble into therapy, and so slowly—how lucky I was—I began to see that the things that were most distressing as I moved through my young adulthood *barely existed outside my head.* It cannot be underrated, that ability to distinguish between outside and in. Left and right I was distorting external realities to make them match my earliest internal ones, or involving myself with people who confirmed old and sorry expectations, or unconsciously cajoling others into buttressing my most unpleasant fears. Neurotic misery, Freud called it. Condemning the future to death so it can match the past, the singer-songwriter Aimee Mann called it. Dr. Aronoff, influenced primarily by the Freud protégée Melanie Klein, called it clinging to the bad breast. Over and over together we found evidence of this insistent grasp. With time I understood that the way I had come to see the world, my place in it, was more about perspective than any absolute reality, and if that was true, at least many more things were possible. I had never been religious, but for the first time in those years I knew what it felt like to believe absolutely in something intangible, to have faith, though Dr. Aronoff made no claims of divinely sanctioned insight. It was simply an education, allied to a temperament more patient than my own, that had allowed her to bestow her gifts. To be able to offer others what she had given me, some freedom from old bad feeling, I just had to go to school, nothing I hadn't done before.

In terms of formal education, several options were available to me on the road to becoming a psychotherapist. The simplest, because of its relative brevity, would have been social work school, but having spent many years listening to my mother lament that social workers got no respect (another masochist's mantra), I was not about to sign up for that. The most lucrative was likely to be medical school, which would set me up to become a psychiatrist, but psychiatrists were no longer necessarily trained in talk therapy: instead, they prescribed pills. I had nothing against medication, but I did not find it interesting in any but the most cursory way. A doctoral program in psychology—comprising four years of theoretical course work and concurrent talk therapy with actual patients, followed by a yearlong clinical internship—seemed like the obvious choice. Dr. Aronoff was neutral but supportive. I half wished for her to tell me she thought I would be good at what she did, but I was well schooled enough by then in the ways of therapy to know we would only examine this desire. For her to explicitly say so would have felt superficial in the context of our relationship anyway, and also less powerful than the fact that in my heart I believed she felt it, as she had for many years been my stalwart teacher.

The first patient I ever saw in therapy had a problem with a kitten. A nineteen-year-old undergraduate at the same university where I was by then in the second year of my doctoral training, she had recently adopted this kitten and had found herself faced with the terrifying realization that she was not responsible enough to care for the animal. She was distraught, really in a panic. Could she simply return it, she wondered, or was it destined to become a victim of her reprehensible immaturity? "He would be so much better off with somebody else," my patient told me with fierce passion as tears stained her translucent skin.

I don't remember how the issue was resolved, if the kitten stayed or went. What I do recall vividly is that my patient and the young cat had some striking autobiographical similarities. Like her pet, my patient had been stuck with a nineteen-year-old single mother, one too irresponsible to parent her to boot. My patient had silently endured her mother's unpreparedness, waiting for what had felt like lifetimes in front of schools or friends' houses for a woman who'd promised earlier that day to pick her up, or in bed for her mother, who she always feared dead, to relieve yet another late-night babysitter. To cope, my patient, like every child before her, honed psychological defenses: ways one protects oneself from anxiety and grief and injuries to self-esteem. She spent many hours lining up her dolls—not playing, just arranging.

While I listened to my patient lament for her poor cat, I knew for certain that she was re-creating an earlier emotional experience of her own, trying the whole scenario out on the kitten to see what would happen. Psychologists call this particularly creative defense "acting out"—replaying once terrifying situations to transform old feelings of vulnerability into experiences of power. Acting out is driven by the unconscious need to master anxiety associated with old and powerfully upsetting fears. We act out what we cannot allow ourselves to remember, and usually even once we've remembered, we forget again and do the whole thing over. Psychologists call this forgetting "repression," the doing over "working through." When viewed from a therapist's chair, it's rather like watching a play in which the star is also writer and director for an unsuspecting supporting cast. By the time I'd met my first patient and heard about her cat, I had read papers on "the repetition compulsion" and "core conflictual relationship themes" and so on and so forth, but I also knew firsthand what it was like to feel so unconsciously compelled to repeat. My own mother's explosiveness had early on left me with two rotten choices: either she was very crazy, or I was very bad. A fair portion of my early adulthood was spent trying to work out which it was, and to that end I befriended more than a couple of high-strung girls, each of whom I grew close to and then finally cut off abruptly, exclaiming "She's crazy!" to anyone who had patience enough to listen. Dr. Aronoff finally asked whom I actually thought I was trying to get rid of.

"When you listen to yourself talk about this cat, *does it remind you of anything*?" I asked my patient cryptically in our early days together. Of course it did not. It was too soon. She was not yet ready to know. Later, as invariably happens, she would re-create an aspect of her childhood dilemma with me, regularly missing sessions as I waited bereft in my office, longing for her to appear just as she'd once ached for her mom. A good therapist uses her own emotional reactions to help the patient put her early experience into words, but I wasn't there yet.

"The unconscious doesn't know who is abandoning whom," one supervisor said to me, explaining that my patient was likely feeling left by me, even though she was the one who was not showing up.

"If she had come regularly and had experienced you as a consistent part of her life, she would have had to grieve all that she didn't have as a child," one of my professors commented in my final weeks of school when I presented the case—which had by that time spanned three years.

I saw many clinic patients during my four years in graduate school. They arrived with their problems and their stories, and because I was being educated in the psychoanalytic tradition, I learned to begin by asking myself two questions. First, what was their developmental level? At what point in their emotional development had things begun to go awry—the earlier it had been, the worse off they were. Second, what was their character organization? In what ways did they tend to distort reality in an attempt to feel less pain? Together these answers provided an important if gross starting point for every treatment. A patient's developmental level was psychotic, borderline, or neurotic; his character organization within that level masochistic or obsessive or narcissistic or depressive—the list goes on some—depending on the constellation of defenses he tended to favor. (Myself, I was neurotic, and my own character style a tinge masochistic with stronger undercurrents of depressive: having felt from quite a young age that painful experiences with my parents were my fault, I believed I was so bad. I was not unlike other psychotherapists in that regard. What better way to alleviate a constant and nebulous sense of guilt than to devote one's life to helping others?)

These two dimensions shed light on the patient's internal experience, on how he organized and perceived his life. What had become more popular in the world at large, under the rubric of cognitive-behavioral therapy, or CBT, was an emphasis on discrete symptoms, say social phobia or panic attacks, that could supposedly be alleviated in short, rote bursts of ten sessions or fewer. At my school patients came to us for long-term work and character change, to alleviate troubling thoughts and behaviors and then some, as true well-being is more than just the absence of symptoms.

In class, semester after semester, we worked our way through a hundred years of psychoanalytic theory in the order it was written. Outside class I sat with patients and supervisors and tried to figure out how to apply my book learning to my clinical work—the most difficult part of becoming a therapist. As I relaxed through those years into the reassurance of my teachers' formulations about the people who arrived to see me weekly, I came to grasp why I had finally chosen to study psychology. Having early on found myself in a world where the attitudes of others confused and pained me, I needed badly to make sense of people, to order them, like my patient with her dolls.

But it was not an auspicious moment for nuanced thought, and while I did not fully realize it yet in those first years of graduate school, neither was it a good time for psychology as a field. As if the pernicious hostility toward the psychoanalytic way of working were not enough to threaten the best chance people had for richer lives, the confluence of cultural forces, the advent of pharmaceutical commercials, and a general human aversion to deep consideration of complication had over the course of many decades swayed the conventional wisdom: psychological problems were nothing more than chemical occurrences in the brain, something one caught, like a cold, or was born with, like color blindness. If Descartes's four-hundred-year-old error had been the separation of mind and body, of rationality and emotion, the modern equivalent, at least in the popular consciousness, seemed to be a separation between brain and mind, in some cases leading to the disappearance of the mind altogether. The medical establishment did not dismiss talk therapy completely, but it seemed to have come to believe that its primary utility was not to make meaning but rather to convince people to take their pills. ("You do the hard work of getting people to be medication compliant," a psychiatry resident said to me once, in the patronizing tone I would become accustomed to hearing from young psychiatrists, as if this were a skill that one might reasonably spend many years in school acquiring.) The sensible idea that the sum total of one's biology *and* life experiences contributed to emotional strengths and vulnerabilities seemed to vanish into air, and along with it esteem for the actual hard work done by psychologists. And so it came to pass that my discipline was slowly being phased out of medical centers—the treatment site of choice for the most disturbed and outcast patients. By the time I completed my four years of doctoral course work and accepted the internship offered me at Kings County Hospital, there were fourteen psychiatrists running and medicating the seven adult inpatient units. There were four psychologists in total covering those wards. Even in the place where I had been invited to complete my training, there was this suggestion of how little what I had to offer might be valued. For my own part, I couldn't quite get that message out of my mind.

- - - - - - - - -

On the first morning of my internship at Kings County Hospital my stomach felt raw. My new professional clothes, so chic in Macy's dressing room just one month before, looked now only dowdy and overly beige. I met my friend Jen on the corner of Joralemon and Court Streets, halfway between our Brooklyn apartments—mine in tree-lined Brooklyn Heights, where I was renting a small fifth-floor walk-up with my classmate turned fiancé, George; Jen's in a grittier, hipper neighborhood just the other side of the Brooklyn-Queens Expressway. We met near the Court Street station to ride the Number 2 train out to the far end of our borough, to East Flatbush, where our Jewish immigrant relatives might have settled just two or three generations prior, but which was now home to other, darker-skinned newcomers: Haitians, Jamaicans, Trinidadians, Guyanese. It was less than five miles from where I'd lived for years, but until I interviewed at the hospital, I'd never as much as passed through the neighborhood. In a city of destinations, East Flatbush was not one at all.

Jen, as of that day my fellow intern, had been my friend for six years, since we'd met in a group therapy class when beginning the master's degrees that we hoped would make us competitive doctoral applicants. We worked in the same research lab, and though she thought of herself as painfully shy, we'd slipped straightaway into an effortless friendship. I grew so attached to her during the two years of our M.A. work that I cried when we didn't get into the same Ph.D. program. "Maybe we'll go on internship together," she said at the time, trying to cheer me. But internship was far off enough then to be only an abstraction, and winding up with Jen seemed unlikely besides. With so many different sites in New York City alone, it was doubtful we would pick the same one, let alone that one would agree upon us. But as we had discussed our respective preference lists just before Match Day that past February, it turned out that both of us—ready for a gritty challenge—had put Kings County in slot number two. Both of us had been certain we wouldn't get the other public hospitals that had been our first picks.

Jen's clothing that morning matched mine, in broad sweeps, and looked equally as labored. We had to appear professional now, business casual. Even the moniker was unattractive. "How are you feeling?" she asked.

"Ambivalent," I answered as we chose seats on the near-empty subway car of our reverse commute. Jen smiled, which I'd known she would do because it was a psych-grad-student inside half joke, the obligatorily measured response of one under constant press to demonstrate how in touch she is with her mixed feelings. In actuality, I was more rueful than anything. While we were still technically students, I knew we'd never be returning to campus again. I was thirty-four years old, and certainly it was time, but I'd loved almost everything about graduate school and could think of little benefit to its end. I enjoyed dividing my time between reading and seeing patients, and discussing the readings and the patients with people who were just as interested in it all as I was. I was living on student loans, which, supplemented by the occasional writing assignment, provided for the basics. And then there was the security inherent in the student position, the absence of any pressure to be the final word.

"Was George excited this morning?" she asked.

Yes, I nodded, he was. As Jen and I traveled farther out into Brooklyn, George, whom I would marry in the spring, was on his way into Manhattan to begin his own internship at Columbia-Presbyterian, the most coveted of placements—a private hospital affiliated with an Ivy League university—and one that hadn't even seen fit to grant me a second interview last winter when the whole matching process was in bloody swing. George had been a social worker in the navy before he'd gone back to school, and he'd struggled over whether to rank Columbia over one of the three local VA hospitals, but in the end he couldn't resist the siren call of the world-class medical institution. Geographically, Columbia was about as far as you could get from Kings County within the borders of New York City. It seemed like an apt metaphor.

The train rumbled down the tracks. Speaking over its clatter, Jen told me she was already wishing the year away. Like many of her classmates, she'd worked at Beth Israel for three years during grad school (we called these placements externships), and she'd had enough of hospitals. Most of my own classmates had also done hospital externships during school, but I'd purposely avoided that, choosing to train at a psychoanalytic institute instead, with healthier patients and different objectives. I'd been halfheartedly cautioned against this by my school's externship adviser—he spoke vaguely about the value of having hospital experience pre-internship—but all of my professors were psychoanalysts in private practice, grooming us for much of the same. I wanted to get right into it. This other work seemed like a lesser option, a booby prize. During my master's program I had briefly volunteered on an inpatient psychiatric unit in order to build my CV, and I believed I'd learned nothing. I'd helped the handlebar-mustachioed recreation therapist run groups, which meant sitting with him and the patients as we put together a unit newsletter (he eventually left me alone to run that group, thanks—but no thanks—to my magazine background) or played hangman, cautiously renamed Wheel of Fortune by the staff. In my semester there I never once encountered a psychologist. Now, some years of training later, I still had no idea what therapists like me, schooled in long-term recovery with higher-functioning patients, were supposed to do in places aimed at short-term stabilization of the chronically and acutely mentally ill. I felt too embarrassed to ask, half-certain that after six years in school I should know that already and half-afraid that the answer would simply validate the fear that I was superfluous.

The alarm bells of the subway station's emergency exit gate blared as Jen and I disembarked at the front of the train. I'd exited subway stations throughout the sprawling city over many years but never to the sound of sirens. I assumed they were meant to summon the police, but nobody came. There didn't seem to be an emergency anyway. Jen and I climbed the stairs into a sunny July morning. We walked straight toward the BP station, left as the road dead-ended at the hospital's A Building, and right down Winthrop Street a good long way.

In 1831, the population of Flatbush hovered around a thousand, and Brooklyn was a city in its own right. That year the medical facility that would grow into Kings County Hospital opened as a one-room infirmary. Over a century, it became the third-largest medical center in the United States, its collection of buildings in ugly juxtaposition, their unseemly mix of architectural styles spread over twenty-four acres of flat city land. The G Building arrived with World War II. Its Gothic architecture suited its label: insane asylum. Of course no one called it that anymore—now it was Behavioral Health—but it was still an asylum in the popular imagination. My intern class would be the last to both begin and end its tenure in G. A new, $120 million facility for psychiatric patients was scheduled to open a year and a half after my start date.

When I arrived there in the summer of 2007, the decaying G Building's seven floors housed 230 psychiatric inpatients when filled to capacity, which was more or less always. Its first floor held administrative offices, a small deli window where staff or visitors could buy coffee and sandwiches, and CPEP— the Comprehensive Psychiatric Emergency Program, more commonly known as the psych ER. The second floor was home to a pharmacy and, without irony intended, a unit dedicated to "dual diagnosis" patients, those with co-occurring substance abuse problems and mental illness. The third, fourth, and fifth floors were each home to two locked general wards. The sixth floor had once been for forensic inpatients—men and women convicted of crimes and also in need of treatment for psychiatric problems. The serial killer Son of Sam had been incarcerated there for a time in the late 1970s. No patients had resided there, though, since Kings County's forensic unit had merged with Bellevue's in Manhattan some years back, and now the cavernous sixth floor was almost deserted, a dimly lit ghost town with a big empty space for meetings, a handful of offices for staff, and one dank room for the seven adult interns to share. On the seventh floor was a bare-bones gym where patients who were well enough could supposedly get some exercise. Though the building was cleaned regularly and thoroughly, it appeared almost filthy, the years of grime and bad feeling having finally worked their way into the linoleum and the concrete.

Jen and I walked through the back door of G to wait for the elevator that would take us to the sixth floor. The elevator system—which we had been introduced to when we came for our internship interviews six months prior—was arcane. The call buttons didn't work, and like so many problems in G they must have been deemed unfixable because the hospital had hired elevator operators to run each lift. To let the operator know you needed to go up or down, you had to pound on the metal door, shouting "one," or whatever floor number you happened to be calling from. If the elevator operator—usually perched on a stool inside the shaft reading the *Post* or texting or selling knockoff designer handbags, depending on who was working that shift—happened to hear you, you would be granted your ride, as long as the operator could get his or her car to actually stop at your floor. (Sometimes the buttons inside the elevators didn't work either, and the operator would yell "I'll be back" as he glided past.) The inpatient units and the stairwells were locked and unlocked with old-fashioned skeleton keys—five inches of nickel-plated steel and heavy in the hand—and the staff took advantage of their cartoon-ish bulk to make the necessary ruckus on the elevator doors. By six weeks into the year, all of us interns were quite fond of the elevator operators, who greeted our trainee eagerness with almost equal enthusiasm each morning. I asked someone on staff what would happen to the operators once Behavioral Health moved to the $120 million building. "They'll still run the elevators," said the person quizzically. Had anyone ever been so new to Kings County Hospital as I?

Jen and I arrived on the sixth floor and walked toward its rotting main space. Streamers hung limply from the ceiling tiles over bagels and tubs of whipped butter and plastic cutlery. An air-conditioning unit—suspended in one of the room's wall of Gothic-looking windows with their grids of rusting panes—cooled the large room. A sign on the wall, left over from the previous week, bade the outgoing intern class fare-well. I envied that group, so far ahead of me in their training. I didn't know any of them personally, though Jen had received and shared what felt like a carefully worded e-mail from one a couple months prior, a response to some questions Jen had sent her about the internship. The e-mail warned about the lack of amenities like toilet paper in the sixth-floor bathrooms, department politics, and the new director of training, who had started midway through the previous interns' time there: "I think Dr. Brent will come into his own during your year, so you'll get to watch him develop, but don't be afraid to stand up for what you want and demand changes, especially when things get out of control."

The place was filled with Behavioral Health staff who'd been summoned to greet us. For morning, the mood was festive. Staff introduced themselves sleepily to us as they ate. The interns gathered in a circle, ten of us, seven adult track and three child. We were demographically representative of our discipline: eight women and two men. All in our early to mid-thirties. Five of the women were Jewish, and two of those Israeli. One of the women was black and one a native Spanish speaker. Intern classes all over the city looked just like us, though most sites did not have quite as many trainees.

Of the six other adult interns, I had known two for years, Jen and Leora, who had been my classmate in graduate school. Friendly if never quite friends, we were the only two of our class of sixteen to be on internship together, the others spread throughout the city and up the East Coast. We hugged in greeting, not having seen each other since classes ended in May. The others introduced themselves in turn: Zeke in an odd corduroy suit with elbow patches, Tamar with a terrible cold, Alisa bubbly and pretty, Bruce curly-haired and wry. The child-track interns said hello, too, though with slightly less interest, as we weren't sure how much to invest in each other, how much our time there might intersect.

As we all exchanged information, our director of training appeared in our circle, though I hadn't seen him approach. Scott, as he would instruct us to call him, would never seem to walk into a room, but rather simply to manifest, a desultory rabbit from a long-battered hat. "Welcome," he said, spreading his arms in front of him. He was average height and slender, boyish, though certainly well past forty, with thinning blond hair and a sallow complexion. There was warmth in his voice, but it was tinged with an irony that negated it, the armor of a man eager to convey that he didn't want us to imagine that he took himself—this role—too seriously. "I've met all of you except . . . well, you must be Darcy, and you must be Zeke. Glad to finally lay my own eyes on you two."

Though it was customary for intern applicants to interview for internships with the director of training, Scott Brent had not yet taken over the job when I'd first set foot on the grounds of the hospital the previous December, early in the interview process. Kings County had actually been my first interview, and after waking up at 3:00 a.m. in a panic and not falling back to sleep (internship is a necessary precursor to finishing the degree, and that year, nationally, there were only spots available for 75 percent of applicants), I became one of the first interviewees of the season to arrive there. My timing meant that I interviewed with Sylvia Goldberg, the longtime, beloved director of training, known by that time to be retiring. She and I had clicked instantly. "What's your biggest weakness as a therapist?" she'd asked.

"I'm in a hurry for my patients to get better, and I go too fast," I'd told her.

"Are you working on that?" she replied, looking intensely into my eyes.

"Yes," I assured her, inspired by her earnestness and her gravity of tone.

Dr. Goldberg invited me to come back the following month to meet Dr. Brent, who would after all be the person I reported to directly were I to match at Kings County. "It's your choice," she said. "It won't impact your chances here either way." I did not go back. The trip seemed too far. I didn't think it mattered who the director of training was. Kings County's internship had a good reputation around my graduate program, and that was enough for me. When Scott sent an e-mail in late May to invite me out to the hospital to meet him before my start date, I was more reluctant to say no, not wanting to offend him. But I was fact-checking at a magazine in Times Square in the weeks leading up to internship, and the hour-plus commute would have meant a good three hours away from the office, a hundred dollars out of my paycheck. About to embark on a year of low wages—Kings County called what it paid us a "stipend," not even a salary—I pushed aside my sense that the trip might be a worthwhile investment.

Scott asked for silence in the room, and the psychologists who lingered stopped their conversations so our director could say a few words. "On behalf of the staff of the Behavioral Health department, I want to welcome our new group of trainees to Kings County Hospital," he said, raising his orange juice glass. "We are delighted to have you here. We know that while the year may be a challenging one, we also trust that its rewards will outweigh its difficulties.

"We convened the staff here today because these are the people who will supervise and support you as the year goes on. I can almost guarantee that there is nothing you will experience on the job that someone in this room has not gone through, and they are available to you to lean on, if you should want that along the way. So, thank you all for coming this morning. Behavioral Health, please join me in welcoming this excellent group." The people in the room raised their cups toward us in a friendly gesture, and a few people clapped. We smiled and nodded in response.

When breakfast ended, Scott and Dr. Reemer, the child-track director of training, sat the ten of us down to tell us how our first two weeks would go. We would fill out the tall stack of paperwork required by the hospital, we would meet with the head of each department in Behavioral Health to decide for certain which two elective rotations we wanted to choose (two were elective, and two—inpatient and psych ER—were mandatory), and we would attend a five-day hospital orientation, which Scott described as an incredible waste of a week but one that he had been unable to get us out of. Our training proper, it seemed, would not get under way for a full fourteen days, counting weekends and the Fourth of July. Once it did, our schedules would be packed, he told us, with more than we would be able to keep up with. Rotations in the mornings, and seminars, supervisions, and outpatients in the afternoons. We'd each see two outpatients and run at least one outpatient group, with forty-five minutes of supervision for every forty-five minutes of therapy. Seminars—on topics ranging from psychopharmacology to brief psychotherapy—would each last around ten weeks, with the exception of the neuropsychology and multicultural courses, which would run all year.

"I also want to say a few words about the lawsuit," Scott added. "You probably all saw the headlines in the spring. In response to the suit, the Justice Department will be arriving midwinter to do an investigation, and there will be some changes being made around here in preparation for that visit. None of that will have anything to do with you. Your training will not be impacted, and you shouldn't give any of it a second thought."

The lawsuit, instigated by New York State's Mental Hygiene Legal Service, had been in the local tabloids for a couple months. I'd first heard about it from my classmate Adrienne. She had done an externship at Kings County during our second year of school, and the most telling thing she had to say about it was that she'd noted, as her time there wore on, that she began to take markedly less and less care with her appearance. In May she'd e-mailed me a link to a *New York Post* article titled "B'klyn Psych Ward a Horror Show":

> *The psychiatric ward at Kings County Hospital is a Dickensian nightmare where patients sleep on urine-covered floors, are beaten, and are forcibly injected with mind-altering drugs, according to a shocking lawsuit.*
>
> *The suit, filed in Brooklyn federal court this week, describes horrifying conditions in the emergency and inpatient psych center, known as Building G, where patients are beaten with metal batons, bugs crawl over sleeping bodies, and the bathrooms are rarely cleaned. . . .*
>
> *Patients in Building G often wait for days in a cramped, dirty room for initial evaluations, the suit alleges. At night, they fight for beds, the losers often sleeping on a floor that may "be stained with blood or urine."*
>
> *Patients tread a "treacherously thin line" between demanding basic care and being viewed as "difficult," which could earn "severe and harrowing" consequences, the suit claims.*
>
> *"Raising one's voice or complaining about the unbearable conditions can result in an injection or being strapped to a gurney," the suit claims.*

Consistent with the *Post*'s style, the article's hyperbole made it hard to take seriously. But Scott's outright dismissal of the whole thing felt just as off. I hadn't finished my degree yet, but I was already much too far along not to think about the suit's allegations like a psychologist. My training had taught me there was a grain of metaphorical truth in even the most psychotic of fantasies. I also knew that no one in any given system—be that a family, a corporation, or a hospital— remains untouched by the problems of the larger group. With his emphatic need to preempt any concerns we might have had, it seemed to me that Scott was communicating something else altogether: if our experiences there were to go awry, well, certainly he didn't want to know about it.

Later, over lunch at a pizza place, we interns reassured one another—after all, we'd toured the wards when we interviewed—that things couldn't be as bad as the tabloids alleged. A couple of the interns introduced the concern that the investigation might cost the hospital's training program its accreditation, but soon enough we moved on to matters of greater importance to us, such as which electives we were going to choose, and also a general getting to know one another. For the next week, our group dragged ourselves around Kings County's campus to hear about the rotations we could choose from. The week after that, we sat wordlessly together through a thirty-five-hour hospital orientation that covered topics like hazardous waste disposal and how to avoid sexually harassing anyone. ("I'm a heavy-chested woman," our orientation leader informed the hundred new employees in the room through her microphone. "If someone mentions that, it's sexual harassment!")

During those first two weeks my intern group would share the frustrations of people eagerly waiting to get started with something. My irritation grew each night when I came home to George's stories about his days, quickly filling up with gratifying learning experiences—outpatient therapy with grad students, supervision with big-name psychologists not otherwise employed by the hospital who volunteered their time for the auspicious privilege of affiliation with Columbia-Presbyterian. George had been provided a desk, a computer, and a phone in a proper office he shared with just one of his fellow interns, who also had her own desk, computer, and phone. In this office, he told me offhandedly, there was a private bathroom. (With this pronouncement—he knew all seven Kings County adult-track interns shared one room, you could barely call it an office—I gave him a look, and he proceeded to inform me that, also, the toilet was gold plated.) As he and I went back and forth over whose turn it was to walk the dog, I wondered silently whether Kings County Hospital had been the best second choice.

In the end, Scott Brent and I would agree on only a few things: there was a lot of paperwork to do in those first days, the internship would indeed become demanding, and hospital orientation—other than being a study in the endemic absurdity of bureaucracy—was a complete waste of time. On other matters, it would be harder to see eye to eye.

CHAPTER TWO

I CHOSE FORENSIC PSYCHOLOGY AS MY FIRST ROTATION, though I had absolutely no idea, and by that I mean none whatsoever, just what it might entail—my imaginings about it culled from all the movies I had ever seen (many) and all the television shows I had ever watched (more) that featured cops and criminals. I'd also found myself wanting to work with Dr. Sheldon Wolfe, Kings County forensic psychologist, since I'd interviewed for the internship with him the previous winter. Dr. Wolfe was in his mid-sixties and salty, short and trim and bald. He was a study in contradictions: an Orthodox Jew with a Ph.D. but the demeanor of an Irish policeman. He half reminded me of my father—the first in his family to go to college—his similar gruff mannerisms and too frequent use of the double negative preempting his education like a disclaimer. During our half hour together, Dr. Wolfe and I had talked about detective novels and police procedurals. Ours was the first interview of many I sat through that winter, and the ones that followed were predictable letdowns. Tell-me-about-your-dissertation-research. Why-did-you-decide-to-become-a-psychologist. If the rest of the forensics staff were like Dr. Wolfe, I figured I'd enjoy learning to do whatever it was they did.

As it turned out, forensic psychology encompassed all sorts of things, most of them having to do with evaluation rather than treatment. Who knew? The forensic psychologists at Kings County spent the bulk of their time doing fitness-to-stand-trial evaluations, working not out of the hospital but in a small office on the thirteenth floor of the criminal courthouse in downtown Brooklyn. They called it the court clinic.

Fitness to stand trial concerns a defendant's state of mind leading up to his day in court. Anyone who cannot participate in his own defense in a meaningful way is not fit to be tried. The evaluations work like this: If a defendant seems markedly bizarre—as around 60,000 arrestees annually do—it is the mandate of his attorney, or that of the judge, to refer him for a psychological evaluation. This evaluation is conducted by some combination of two psychologists or psychiatrists and is also called a competency assessment, or a 7:30. The meaningful participation required of the accused may or may not be impaired by any number of psychological problems. After a detailed interview, the investigators write brief reports that end with recommendations to the judge as to the defendant's fitness. Ninety percent of the time, the judge goes along with the clinicians' recommendations. If found unfit, a defendant is treated at a state hospital with medication until he becomes able to understand and make decisions about his charges. If a defendant never becomes fit and the crime is egregious enough, the state can petition to have him committed to an institution in lieu of trying him. For misdemeanors, a defendant may simply be released for time served after his hospitalization has run its course.

The logistics of the forensic rotation would be different from all the others, Scott explained. I would spend two full days a week at the court clinic, while the other interns would be at their various stations Monday through Friday and only in the mornings. It wasn't clear to me how I was supposed to fill the other three mornings, and Scott would only vaguely say that I'd eventually have plenty to do.

On the first day of my forensic rotation, I met Dr. Katherine Young, director of the Brooklyn court clinic and my rotation supervisor, not at the courthouse, but instead at Bellevue Hospital in Manhattan. Kings County and Bellevue were both city hospitals managed by the Health and Hospitals Corporation. Of the two, from what I understood, Kings County was considered the ugly stepchild and held in much lower esteem. In a largely Manhattan-centric city, it had the misfortune to be located at the outskirts of an outer borough, in a neighborhood beset by violent crime. (Army reservists training to be battlefield medics spent time in Kings County's ER and ICU to become accustomed to the trauma wounds— from gunshots and stabbings—they would see once deployed.) Because Kings County no longer housed a forensic ward, prisoners charged with or convicted of crimes in Brooklyn who needed psychiatric hospitalization were sent to Bellevue, but the fitness-to-stand-trial evaluations of the Brooklyn accused were still conducted by the Kings County staff, and so we were in Manhattan on that July Thursday.

Dr. Young was waiting for me in the enormous airy lobby. She was slim and bespectacled, with gray hair, and in her mid-forties. Immediately chatty, she told me that she'd been a professional opera singer before earning her doctorate at Penn State, where she'd become aware of the revolving door between jails and psychiatric hospitals. She decided to commit her life to helping the mentally ill get fair treatment in the justice system. We were at Bellevue that day, she explained, to evaluate three defendants, and we would meet their public defender and another of the forensic psychologists upstairs. As we emerged from a full elevator into the hallway of the locked prison ward, a uniformed guard motioned us to the side. In front of us, a dozen or so shackled black men in orange jumpsuits were being led backward out of a freight elevator. The sight of them was shocking—their shackles and their labored, tandem shuffling. Their jumpsuits were stamped "DOC," for Department of Corrections, in bold letters. Another guard unlocked a metal gate and watched their awkward passing as the rest of us tried to look away.

Dr. Young and I crossed the hallway and entered a waiting room with chairs and a mounted television. She introduced me to the lawyer, Jim Danziger, and the other psychologist, Dr. Pine. The two psychologists conversed happily. Dr. Pine was just back from a long vacation, and they had a lot to catch up on. Jim recognized my Michigan twang from some time he'd spent in Ohio, and he told me about those years. He was truly friendly and we chatted with some energy. Then a guard came and escorted us through the metal gate and another locked door into a small, windowless room with four chairs and a table.

"First we'll see Randall Corbin," Dr. Young told me. "He declined to speak to us once before. He's accused of trying to kill his wife. He keeps writing letters to her, threatening."

"He threatened me, too," said Jim. "Tried to grab me from behind the bars of his cell."

The psychologists decided that Jim should stand near the door. Dr. Young, Dr. Pine, and I would take the chairs. "Do you feel safe?" I asked them. Never having met any, I assumed prisoners were dangerous.

They both replied no, shrugging their shoulders, but neither of them moved. In the end it didn't matter, because Mr. Corbin refused to see us. On the basis of this decision, which they believed reflected paranoia and was not in his best interest, both psychologists would recommend that he be found unfit.

The next defendant was Franklin Drury. He was charged with public indecency. He, too, had threatened Jim, not to kill but to sue him. In the hospital he'd been diagnosed with schizoaffective disorder. I had heard of this but barely knew what it was. The diagnosis came from the *Diagnostic and Statistical Manual*—the *DSM*, which we had not paid much mind to in graduate school, where we were distinctly not being taught to categorize patients according to collections of observable symptoms. In our outpatient clinic we didn't have to: unable to provide the support they needed, we did not see anyone with such debilitating problems. The *DSM* was only a book of lists that I might have sat down and read with some benefit. Between George and me we had two copies. But instead I'd chosen to feel ill at ease in my unfamiliarity with its principles.

Franklin Drury had a long psych history: multiple hospitalizations as well as arrests. The guard asked us to remove some paper clips from the table, and then he brought the prisoner in. Mr. Drury had light brown skin and had twisted some of his locks into braids and knots that made his head look like an unfinished macramé project. In a soothing voice, Dr. Young explained to Mr. Drury why we were there and let him know that our talk was court ordered and therefore not confidential. "Your lawyer believes you're unable to think clearly," she said.

"I've never seen that man," Mr. Drury said, barely glancing at Jim before sharply turning away.

"We've met a few times," Jim corrected him.

"How are you doing here?" asked Dr. Young.

"No one will tell me where I am. They won't give me the address," he said. "I want to let my mother know I'm okay."

"Do you know why you're here?"

He shook his head. "I don't know who, why, or how I got here. I've done nothing to deserve this misery."

"Do you know what you've been charged with?" asked Dr. Pine.

"I don't know for sure," he said.

"Menacing," interjected Jim. "You exposed yourself to two adults and told them you were going to get them, and then you asked two little girls to lift up their skirts."

"I didn't," said Mr. Drury, refusing to look at Jim.

Dr. Young asked some questions to get a sense of our client's history. He was raised by both parents along with an older sister, did okay in school but hadn't had many friends, had gotten through five semesters of college before "some people tried to destroy me. They put drugs in my milk."

"Why would they want to do that?" asked Dr. Young.

"I was studying math, and it was well-known that I was studying," said Mr. Drury. "A girl was investigating the case when I was in college. She turned up dead."

Dr. Young and Dr. Pine scribbled notes. They tried to glean whether Mr. Drury understood basic courtroom procedures and whether he had ideas about how to proceed with his case. He did: he wanted to go to trial. If found guilty, which seemed almost certain, he'd be handed a longer sentence than if he simply took a plea.

"I'm not going to plead out to something I didn't do. I'll testify. How can they not believe me? I'm telling the truth. I don't have time to expose myself to nobody unless it's a woman I like."

"There are witnesses. They may also ask the two little girls to testify," said Dr. Pine. "With your history, why would the jury believe you and not them?"

"People can assert anything, but if they don't have proof, you can't put a person in jail," he said.

"Why would they lie?" asked Dr. Pine.

"I don't know." He stopped to think. "Maybe they're involved with the same people who drugged my milk."

"How likely do you think that is?" she followed up.

"I'm not sure. It's just a guess," he said.

"What kind of sentence do you think you might get if you go to trial?"

"My time has been served," he said.

"No, it hasn't," said Jim.

Mr. Drury could not get past his assertion that he was telling the truth and his belief that if you tell the truth you don't go to jail. Dr. Young and Dr. Pine agreed that his inability to see things more realistically made him unable to understand the likely consequences of choosing to go to trial. For now, they agreed, he was unfit.

Our third defendant of the day was no more the criminal mastermind of my misguided forensic fantasies than the others. A deaf-mute religious Jew, he had communicated in writing to the officers who'd arrested him that he was the terrorist Mohamed Atta, a Pakistani Nazi, and an employee of the Israeli secret police—the modern trinity of a disorganized mind. When Dr. Young asked, with paper and pen, how he wanted to proceed with his charges of menacing, he refused to answer. He would not acknowledge her other questions either.

"This is very important," she wrote to him.

"To you it is very important," he finally scribbled. "To me it is not."

She found him unfit.

When we finished at Bellevue, Dr. Young and Dr. Pine invited me to a late lunch. We ate turkey burgers at a diner on Second Avenue along with an administrator they'd run into in the hospital lobby as we were leaving. The three gossiped about their colleagues, paying cursory homage to the idea that they shouldn't be talking that way in front of an intern. I had no idea whom they were discussing anyway. I'd been happy to be included in their lunch plans, but I felt uncomfortable there, like a girl among men. When lunch ended, Dr. Young said we were finished for the day and that I should go home. As I left the group to take the subway back to Brooklyn alone, Dr. Young put her hand on my forearm with some urgency. "You should always carry ID," she told me. "And if you ever get arrested, don't say anything to the police."

I did jury duty once, in the 1990s, when I lived in Manhattan. The courthouses there are regal, with marble pillars and careening stairways. The Brooklyn criminal courthouse was disappointing in comparison. It looked like any modern office building. On my first morning at the court clinic, I waited before the lobby's metal detectors, which were preventing throngs of impatient visitors from making their way to the elevator banks. Dr. Young came in and saw me waiting in the long and slow-moving line. She motioned me toward her and a much shorter queue. "You can go in the employee entrance with your Kings County ID," she told me. We both passed through the staff metal detector and rode the elevator together to the thirteenth floor making small talk. The sleek elevator moved quickly in response to the press of its buttons, and the spotless corridor into which we emerged was cooled by central air-conditioning. Imperious or not, it was much more pleasant than our G Building.

"Today you'll meet the master's-level forensic students," Dr. Young offered. Sometimes she sounded syrupy and like a Texan, although she was a northerner. "That will be nice for you."

We entered the office. It was narrow and colored in neutral tones, with a hallway that ran parallel first to a small waiting area and then to four cubicles followed by a space in the back with some chairs. Five people who looked as if they might be master's-level students were sitting in the chairs, and after Dr. Young waved at them and entered her office—the only self-contained space in the clinic—I introduced myself as the new psychology intern. They were duly impressed. The career options for master's-level forensic psychologists being limited, they were all contemplating doctoral programs themselves. They asked me where I went to school and wanted to know something about it. When I told them my program's theoretical orientation was psychoanalytic, they looked at me as if waiting for a punch line. They were very young, these students from the John Jay College of Criminal Justice, and most of them lived in the far reaches of almost suburbia with their parents. I guessed from the fact that I was expected to sit with them that our roles at the court clinic would not diverge.

I had finished all of my doctoral course work, for God's sake, and yet here I was stuck beside the master's students. It felt like a demotion.

With the arrival of Dr. Wolfe my mood improved. I said hello and reintroduced myself, reminding him that we'd met the previous winter when he'd interviewed me. He said he remembered and welcomed me to the court clinic before announcing to the group that he would be teaching the Tuesday seminar, which was apparently a weekly occurrence. That morning he would talk about the history of the fitness to stand trial.

Forensic psychology textbooks trace the idea of fitness to stand trial back to seventeenth-century England. In those days, criminal defendants who refused to respond to the charges against them were given a sort of pretrial during which a jury would decide whether they were "mute of malice" or "mute by visitation of God." The first verdict decreed them willfully obstreperous and was met with physical punishment that could end only upon response to the charges or death. The second initially applied to the physiologically deaf and mute but was eventually broadened to include the lunatic. The lunatic, forgiven his silence, was exempt from torture.

While the textbooks talked about the seventeenth century, Dr. Wolfe explained that he located the origins of competency in the year 200 and the Talmudic concept of the *shoteh*. The *shoteh* displayed disorganized thinking and behavior. He was exempt from following Jewish law, could not enter into a contract, and was exonerated from punishment. With the establishment of the United States, similar ideas came to be loosely reflected in the Constitution, not only to preserve the rights of the individual, but also to avoid making a mockery of the court system, whose players and tasks would certainly lose dignity in the process of trying someone quite obviously out of his mind.

The rights guaranteed criminal defendants by the Constitution had been fleshed out over time, and so, too, the definition of fitness to stand trial. The U.S. Supreme Court, Dr. Wolfe told us, established the modern-day competency standard in 1960 with *Dusky v. United States.* Milton Dusky—a thirty-three-year-old chronic schizophrenic accused of being an accessory to the kidnapping and rape of a teenage girl— was initially deemed competent by a judge whose own standard was simply that a defendant be oriented to person, time, and place (that is, know who he is, when it is, and where he is). The justices later overturned Dusky's conviction on the grounds that this judge's idea of fitness was incomplete and that Dusky, whose psychiatrist had observed that he was unable "to interpret reality from unreality," had not indeed been fit to stand trial. The Court established that "the test must be whether [the defendant] has sufficient present ability to consult with his lawyer with a reasonable degree of rational understanding—and whether he has a rational as well as factual understanding of the proceedings against him." Once treated and found fit according to these standards, Dusky was retried and reconvicted, though with a much lighter sentence the second time around.

Dr. Wolfe told us that in 1974 the New York courts had elaborated on the *Dusky* standard, requiring that a defendant meet six basic criteria in order to be found fit. The first three were relatively easy to ascertain. A defendant must know who he is, where he is, and when it is, or be, as the jargon goes, "oriented in all spheres." He must be able to perceive, recall, and relate—to communicate effectively about his life and the world and about the charges against him. He must be able to understand the role of the court principals and procedures, at minimum knowing or being able to learn what a judge and jury do.

The second three criteria were less black-and-white, leaving room for debate among assessors. A defendant must be able to establish a working relationship with his attorney. He must be able to choose rationally among the various legal alternatives available to him and to understand the possible outcomes and consequences of each choice. Finally, he must be sufficiently emotionally stable to maintain coherence throughout the stressful process of a trial. Varying widely across jurisdictions, anywhere between 1.2 and 77 percent of those referred for competency evaluations are found unfit. Dr. Wolfe told us that the Brooklyn forensic team deemed more defendants incompetent than those in any other borough. He was obviously proud of this—of the integrity they brought to the justice system and the protection they provided these defenseless defendants—which made me excited to be a part of it, too.

When Dr. Wolfe finished, he returned to his cubicle. It was still early. "What happens now?" I asked one of the others.

"We wait here," he said. "When the doctors go down to the holding cells, they take us with them, two at a time, to watch."

Dr. Wolfe overheard. "Actually," he chimed in, "I'm going to treatment court this morning. Only one of you can come. Any takers?" I had never heard of treatment court, and I did want to go but wasn't sure what the etiquette was in the group. I waited, though not very long, to see whether anyone else volunteered. When no one did, I stood up, and Dr. Wolfe and I made our way out of the office to ride the elevator downstairs.

Was I expected to know what treatment court was? Was I supposed to have any idea whatsoever about forensic psychology? I'd figured the rotation would expose me to a branch of my field I knew nothing about, but was that also the expectation that the rotation had of me? I must have looked uneasy because Dr. Wolfe asked, "Everything going okay?"

"Yes," I said, but then decided to lay it all on the line, my inexperience and inadequacy: "So what is it we're doing this morning? What is treatment court?"

Dr. Wolfe did not look aghast. He explained in his paradoxically good-natured and cantankerous way: "The court recognizes that nonviolent drug offenders aren't necessarily criminally minded but that they commit crimes to support their drug habits. Locking them up doesn't make a whole lot of sense; they're just going to go back to using and crimes that support using as soon as they get out. So they offer an alternative: do a drug treatment program rather than serve jail time. If they complete the program and stay clean for a certain amount of time, the charges are wiped from their record. We're called to evaluate the defendants eligible for treatment court when their lawyers think there might be mental health issues. So the woman we're going to see today, we need to find out, first of all, whether she's interested in a program and, second, if there are psychological issues that need to be addressed in order for her to complete it successfully."

This didn't quite make sense to me, because developing a drug problem was in and of itself evidence of a whole host of messy psychological issues. But I knew I had to shift my thinking according to context. The courts were probably concerned only about the most pronounced psychotic symptoms—hallucinations and delusions and such—and those were what we had likely been called in to assess. I resented having to make this adjustment. It felt like selling out. Still, having little knowledge about or faith in the offerings of the justice system, I was surprised that such a reasonable thing as treatment court existed. I let my bad feeling go and thought instead: fantastic.

The person we sat down across from in a small space adjacent to one of the building's many courtrooms was less enthusiastic. Maria was thirty-nine and frayed. She was Hispanic, pretty if too thin after years of taking in less food than heroin—about two hundred dollars' worth a day, she told us, rolling up her sleeves to show us the track marks on her arm. She was on methadone now. "I wouldn't be able to sit here and have a conversation with you if I wasn't," she told us. She'd started drinking and cutting herself at a young age, soon after her uncle began sexually abusing her, and then an older friend introduced her to heroin, which she eventually began prostituting herself to get, conceiving two children that way. Both were living with their grandmother. Her eyes teared up and she looked ashamed when she told us this, and I felt remorse about being there, an unnecessary interloper on Dr. Wolfe's work. She said she wasn't much interested in a program, and Dr. Wolfe asked why. She answered, "I was the middleman in a drug buy, a B felony. I'll get one to three months. A program is five times that long."

"Sad," I observed as we left. Maria had this traumatic history that she relied on drugs to numb herself against, and she didn't know that therapy might make that numbing less imperative.

Dr. Wolfe agreed. He said he was going to recommend a program rather than jail time despite what she'd said. Maybe she'd take it once she had more time to think. "She's an unusual case," he said. "She seemed reachable." It seemed regrettable that we would not be the ones to try to reach her. On forensics, I quickly got it, we weren't that kind of psychologist.

I went back upstairs with Dr. Wolfe, and we found Dr. Pine, whom I'd met at Bellevue, waiting for him. Dr. Wolfe went to the back to collect one more student, and the four of us plus the lawyer Jim Danziger were off to see another defendant in the basement holding cells where most of their business was conducted. I felt energized by the pace of the morning and all the things I was learning that were new to me. "We're assessing a female defendant today," said Dr. Pine. "Young and charged with assault in the third degree. Grabbed a woman's breasts."

Our group rode the elevator to the lobby and then took a long flight of cement stairs down to a very cold and vast underground complex. We signed in with the guards, went through more metal detectors, and were admitted to a holding cell, a large room painted steel gray with metal bars like a jail cell on a movie set. The female defendant was brought in, no laces in her shoes. The officers uncuffed her before she sat down across from us. Dr. Pine introduced us and explained why we were there. The woman's name was Katrina, and she was nineteen years old and jailed at Rikers Island as she awaited trial. She rocked back and forth on the bench, smiling and looking off to the side as if at someone, though we five were seated across from her. She knew her Social Security number and her birthday and that she'd earned a GED. She also knew that she'd been hospitalized for psychiatric reasons for the first time at age fourteen, by her mother, and that she'd since been readmitted at least fifteen times.

"What are your symptoms?" asked Dr. Wolfe.

"Nausea," she answered.

"Any voices?" he followed up.

"All the time," she said. "They annoy me. Say, 'Katrina did this, Katrina did that.'"

"Are you hearing them now?"

"Yes. I'm trying to figure out how they're there, every-where I go."

"Do you recognize the voice?"

"It's the same person all the time. A lady's voice. Bother-ing me." She looked off to the side again and laughed.

"What's funny?" asked Dr. Pine softly.

Katrina didn't answer.

Jim Danziger—who was not technically required to be there and had very little official business during the course of any evaluation—sat scanning and highlighting an issue of *The New Yorker* as if it were a used textbook. He'd been represent-ing clients like Katrina for longer than I'd been alive, and like Silly Putty laid over newsprint, he bore the stain of their mannerisms. His questions often tumbled out abruptly and in response to stimuli the rest of us were not quite privy to. "So what happened the day you were arrested?" he asked.

"I went to a department store to buy something."

"Why'd you grab this woman?" Jim was less gentle than Dr. Pine and Dr. Wolfe, and I got the sense that while they liked him, they didn't often appreciate his interruptions.

Katrina began laughing again. "She's lying. She's a good liar. She's a lying liar. A good lying liar." Katrina was very fat and wore orange sneakers. Her flesh shook all over as she laughed.

"What do you plan to do about the charge?" asked Dr. Wolfe.

"Fight it," said Katrina.

"What would your defense be?"

"I'd tell the truth."

Dr. Wolfe paused. "So what did happen then?"

"It's like, I just kept passing by her, and she probably thought I was stalking her. She hit me first. It was a fight."

"Do you want to go to trial?" asked Dr. Pine.

Katrina looked off to the side again. She said, "I don't *know* why they're so eager to put me in jail!"

Dr. Wolfe redirected her, and she explained to him her understanding of courtroom procedures and participants. When he praised her, she looked directly at him for the first time before blurting out, "To tell the truth, I do that all the time and walk away!" She went back to laughing with the companion the rest of us could not see. Like the defendants I saw at Bellevue, she was not oriented to reality and would be found unfit.

After that we interviewed two more like her. Both men heard voices, wore shoes rendered laceless to preclude suicide, and could not make logical decisions about how to proceed with their charges. Unfit, unfit. We returned upstairs, and I settled back in the waiting area. The master's students flirted and made boozy weekend plans. By four o'clock the staff was packing up. The defendants had to be taken back to Rikers around three, and once the psychologists' paperwork had been finished, there wasn't anything left to do. I went home to take the dog for a walk along the promenade and wait for George, who had been getting home much later than I. It was our fourth week of internship, and while I was eagerly awaiting the assignment of outpatient cases and supervisors and seminars to fill my days, he was already swamped with work and with classes—five outpatients and five outpatient supervisors, a rotation in a drug and alcohol treatment center, seminars with heady titles. The discrepancy had me antsy, worried that I wasn't going to get enough.

When George got home, I told him about my day: Dr. Wolfe's lecture, treatment court, the basement holding cell. "So all you're supposed to do is watch these interviews for three and a half months?" he asked.

"I guess so," I said, feeling protective of the experience. "But they're interesting. The defendants are basically psychiatric patients, just in a different setting."

"Well, I'm sure that will be good," he said, only almost trying to keep the skepticism out of his voice. It irked me, not least because I quickly made it my own.

George told me about his day. He'd been assigned some interesting cases and was excited about the analytically trained supervisors he'd met so far. At least one of his seminars seemed as if it was going to be thought provoking, as good as any of the best classes we'd shared in the last four years. Columbia-Presbyterian was clearly more like grad school than Kings County. I missed school intensely then—my supervisors, my classes, my patients there. One of the latter had wanted to continue our work together after my course work ended, to come see me at the hospital's outpatient clinic, but in an e-mail exchange over the summer Scott had declined to approve that, suggesting that the very request was indicative of my own pathology—a difficulty coping with separation and loss. (Having your personality critiqued was an expectable part of being a doctoral student in clinical psychology, so it wasn't a particularly surprising rejoinder.) "What about the fact that long-term cases are valuable to your training?" Dr. Aronoff had asked, with feeling, in the last session we had before internship began—logistics would make it impossible for us to meet during the coming year. In her voice I heard the chagrin that might have been my own had I not leaped so quickly to feeling shamed. I tended to take all criticism to heart. It seemed the one true thing.

George's training director had allowed him to transfer one of *his* grad school patients to the outpatient clinic at the Pres (as he and his fellow male interns were calling it, in tones of jaunty Ivy rowers). He had been seeing this old patient since week one of internship, Tuesdays and Thursdays. This was another point in favor of his fancy private hospital—the opportunity to do twice-weekly outpatient treatment. I sighed at my own predictability. Was I bound to spend the whole of the year comparing my experience with George's and always to find my own wanting?

One of my graduate school supervisors once made the offhand remark that a lot of people walk around a little psychotic a lot of the time. I was in my fourth year, and in my inexperience this took me by surprise, though I had by then read enough that it might not have. On forensics what I saw was that, also, a lot of people walk around a lot psychotic a lot of the time. With Dr. Wolfe's lecture on the ambiguity inherent in the fitness standards in mind, I'd looked forward to animated debates about whether this one could make rational choices about his options, or that one could maintain emotional stability throughout a trial. But each of the men and women who sat down across from us in the basement holding cell was simply batshit. It didn't leave much to discuss.

Dedon Willis wore several dirty T-shirts and baggy jeans. At first he was very upset, too agitated to listen to the doctors' questions or take in the charges presented him by his lawyer,

Jim Danziger. "I want this case to be dropped," he insisted over and over, raising his arms and popping off the bench a couple inches, then finally settling down. "I don't know what they said I did."

"Disturbing the peace. Screaming at people on the subway. Spitting on a police car. Cursing out a cop." Jim ran down the list.

"It's not true! This case is garbage. I want to get out of here," he said. He had a black eye after three fights at Rikers. He was homeless with a long history of psych hospitalizations. He was twenty-seven and had been arrested eighteen times.

"The first case you had was serious," said Jim.

"We don't need to go there," said Mr. Willis.

"Attempted murder," Jim told us. "He did four years upstate."

"Why did you scream at those people?" asked Dr. Ruben, one of the two psychiatrists on the forensic staff.

"I woke up on the subway, and I didn't know where I was at," he told us angrily.

"Why did you spit on the police car?"

"The cop was bothering me. He was telling people my business. I told him not to talk about me in public."

Jim cut in. "Better than his last arrest. Last time he tried to punch an officer who bumped into him."

"They're always trying to get under my skin!"

Dr. Pine asked what medication he was on. "Haldol. But I don't take it every day. I don't use drugs. That's why I don't take my medication. It's a drug."

"How do you want to resolve these charges?"

"I want to get out," he said.

"You can either go to trial or take a plea," explained Dr. Ruben.

"Is it a felony or a misdemeanor?" he asked. The latter. "I'm not stupid. Why should I go to trial on a misdemeanor?" Then in the same breath, "I want to go to trial. It's my word against the cop."

The doctors and Jim looked at each other. "It has to be one or the other," said Jim. "My job is to help you decide."

"I'm not talking to you, man." Mr. Willis spit toward Jim's foot. "I'm not stupid. I'm not stupid."

The Brooklyn courthouse was a ten-minute walk from my apartment. I had never before worked so close to home. Had anyone? It was luxurious. I took to buying coffee from the breakfast cart on the corner halfway between home and the office. Soon the guy who ran it knew my order. Milk no sugar.

In the basement holding cell Dr. Wolfe, Dr. Pine, Jim Danziger, a master's student, and I sat waiting. We were a big crowd. On the outside it was still very hot, but the basement might have doubled as a meat locker, and I always brought a sweater. Our first defendant walked in handcuffed and escorted by a guard. He removed her restraints, and she sat down across from us. Her name was Beth. She was white with stringy hair. She was thirty and woozy. Jim announced her charges: assault in the second and third degree. She told us she was living at Rikers and listed the antipsychotic medications she was taking. I was learning the names of drugs that none of my graduate school patients had been on: Risperdal, Seroquel, Abilify, Depakote. They signified serious problems, as if in the holding cell these were ever remotely in question. Beth knew what month it was and the year—she was "oriented to time"—but she told us she had memory problems.

"What kinds of things do you forget?" asked Dr. Wolfe.

"Sometimes my name," she said.

She remembered that she'd been hospitalized for the first time at thirteen.

"How come?" asked Dr. Wolfe.

"I tried to kill myself," she said.

"What was going on?"

"My parents died. Something like that."

Jim sat with his *New Yorker*, highlighting passages in slippery green.

Beth told us she'd been born in the United States but grown up in Haiti, where her parents were missionaries. After they died, she returned to New York, where her aunts and uncles had declined to take her in and she was put into foster care. At nineteen she returned to Haiti, where she met a woman named Joanna who she believed was her sister. Dr. Pine flipped through Beth's chart. "It says here she's obsessed with Joanna," Dr. Pine whispered to Dr. Wolfe, but loud enough for everyone to hear.

"After I met Joanna, other people in my family started dying," Beth told us. "And now sometimes I hear her voice, telling me to do things to people. She told me to attack those women."

"She's delusional," Jim announced, putting down his magazine.

"In the U.S. you call them delusions, but that's not what we call them in Haiti. In Haiti we call it voodoo, and there are laws against it. I want to see a Haitian doctor who can help me with the voodoo and my visions."

"So how about the insanity defense?" Dr. Pine asked our lawyer friend in the same half whisper she'd used before.

"That was my original plan, but she'll get more time in the hospital with that than she will in jail for what she did, so it doesn't make any sense."

"Do you understand what will happen if you go to trial?" asked Dr. Wolfe.

"I'm not going to trial," she said.

"So what is your plan?" he followed up.

"I don't have a plan," she said.

She refused to speak anymore, and the doctors summoned the guard, who cuffed her and escorted her out. Unfit, the doctors agreed.

"Is anyone ever fit?" I asked Dr. Wolfe quietly. I didn't want to embarrass myself with a stupid question. Maybe people were found fit all the time, and I just hadn't seen it yet.

"Sometimes," he said, without lowering his voice. He was as unself-conscious as I was reticent, which was partly why I enjoyed him so much. "But think about who refers them for evaluation—lawyers and judges. Unless it's a lawyer grasping at straws to get his client out of something, they're usually just sending us people who are pretty obviously disturbed. Also, the mentally ill wind up arrested a lot. Twenty-five percent of inmates meet criteria for a psychotic disorder."

Another defendant was brought in. He was twenty-six and from the islands. He was big and looked menacing until he sat down and started to cry fat tears like a toddler's. Dr. Pine and Dr. Wolfe could not establish whether he had a history of psych hospitalizations or had simply been in the hospital for other health problems. The defendant was too confused to be helpful. Not fit. As the guard led him out, I reluctantly got up and excused myself to go back to the hospital. Seminars were starting that week, and though the topics would shift, the timing would not. One month in and my days at forensics were from then on to be interrupted. The hospital was an hour door-to-door from the court clinic, and the seminars were that long as well, so I'd be missing three hours at my rotation to attend them, which made little sense to me, but it was the schedule I'd been handed. Our first mandatory seminar was on group therapy, and at least it was a modality close to my heart. I'd co-led a group for women with eating disorders during my last two years of school, and I'd loved it, the fast pace and the treacly intimacy.

I arrived at the N Building, the child and family clinic, where the seminar was taking place, and I found that our teachers were two junior psychologists not long past internship themselves. In grad school, seasoned psychologists taught and supervised within specific areas of expertise; at Columbia-Presbyterian, too. I'd anticipated the same at Kings County, though I would later wonder if in this expectation I'd only been setting myself up for disappointment. "What is a group?" our teachers proposed once everyone was assembled. "Is a group one person? Is a group two people? Is a group a bunch of strangers waiting in line together at a grocery store?"

We were seated around a large table—the adult-track interns, the child-track interns, and a handful of psychiatry residents whom we'd only seen around. We interns shot each other looks to relieve a strong mutual feeling of insult. We replied to our teachers in silence, a tool of our trade. The psychiatry residents picked up our slack.

"A group can be anything!" exclaimed one of them, a salt-and-pepper-haired man in plastic-framed glasses.

"Groups are everywhere!" offered another with undue enthusiasm. I imagined that there must have been few rhetorical questions in medical school. Maybe they hadn't been allowed to speak at all.

The teachers seemed relieved to have participants. They all went back and forth. An hour passed this way, the interns stony faced, the psychiatry resident with the glasses proudly sharing group techniques he was pioneering, like this one to deal with reticent, inpatient adolescents: "I curse to let them know that I'm cool." We interns told him that if foul language did not come naturally to him, the kids would see right through it. Like most of us seated around the table that afternoon, he looked disheartened.

By the time I made it back to the court clinic in the afternoon, the doctors were already well into their post-lunch interviews in the holding cells downstairs. I couldn't go down to join them, because one could not just waltz into the basement as if arriving at a potluck supper. The conflict between forensics and didactics was obviously going to be a problem. I went to Scott to explain my predicament, suggesting that I occasionally be excused from the Tuesday or Thursday class in order to actually spend the entire day that had been promised me on my rotation. My request seemed so reasonable that it surprised me when he said "Absolutely not" and looked at me with some suspicion, as if I were a high school student trying to wriggle out of last period.

A couple days later, during a meeting where Scott pointed out for the third time in as many weeks that Zeke and I were the only interns he hadn't handpicked (could that have really been such an injurious affront? I refused to believe it), there arose an actual something I wanted to get out of: an unfortunate supervisory assignment. It was for a case in the outpatient clinic. I was assigned to a patient named Carmen Thompson, and Scott announced that I would be supervised by the staff neuropsychologist, Dr. Caitlin Downs. Neuropsychology is a specialty within clinical psychology. Neuropsychologists do testing, not therapy. While Dr. Downs would've had a graduate school education at least marginally similar to my own, she had chosen to specialize afterward in something that had nothing to do with being a therapist and had likely not seen any patients herself since her own internship. All of my supervisors in graduate school had been not only Ph.D. therapists but also psychoanalysts, which meant that they had spent a minimum of five years in intensive postdoctoral therapy training; most of them had decades of experience as practitioners besides. I raised an obvious objection: "But she's a *neuro*psychologist."

Scott was nonplussed. "She's a *licensed* psychologist. That's all that matters here," he said. Jen and Leora made sympathetic faces from across the table. Remembering that two of my classmates had come back from their internship interviews with Scott talking enthusiastically about wanting to be supervised by him, I decided to take one last stab at relieving myself of the non–therapist.

"Do you have any interest in supervising the case?" I asked him, trying to adopt his winking tone. "I've heard you're pretty good."

Scott looked at me with a deep skepticism, his perpetually raised eyebrow, a shake of the head. I'd asked for too many adjustments already, and the asking itself had begun to offend him. I didn't like where that left me, but there was nothing to be done about it. Scott went back to addressing the group.

"You should call your patients to set up your first appointments immediately. The old interns told them to expect to hear from you sometime in August. You'll also need to speak to your supervisors to set up supervision times. Do that as soon as possible, too. Preferably before you see your patients. Your supervisors all worked with the last interns on these cases, so they can give you a heads-up about who you're seeing."

In the midst of all those forensic assessments, I felt pressed to get going with my outpatient work and soon, so I walked down the poorly lit hall to Dr. Downs's office straight after the meeting. She'd already introduced herself as Caitlin in passing, as her office, along with Scott's, flanked the intern room. She and he were the best of friends, constantly dancing back and forth between each other's doorways to speak in conspiratorial whispering verse.

"Your new patient doesn't exactly make therapy a priority," Caitlin said to me as she invited me in. She closed her door and shook her head and made a face. She was probably forty, with blond-tinted hair and airbrushed acrylic nails that said "Queens" to me. I was not much younger, of course, and apparently a snob. "We got her to the point last year where at least she would call when she wasn't coming," Caitlin continued. "You need to let her know from the get-go that she has to give you at least twenty-four hours' notice if she's going to cancel."

Caitlin seemed to want me to join her in her distaste for the patient. Instead, I felt it toward her. Our supervisory relationship no more than two minutes in duration, Caitlin had already said at least three things that offended my sensibilities as a therapist and given me one explicit order that I knew I would not carry out. "If a patient doesn't show up, we call it *resistance*," I wanted to begin, the voice in my head unbearably disdainful. How quickly I disliked myself in her presence.

"What do you think she's communicating in not showing up?" I asked instead. This is one thing my graduate school supervisors would have thought about had they been supervising the case for the last year, but I might have worked harder to get the tone out of my voice.

"Just make sure you let her know she needs to call you in advance," Caitlin reiterated.

There was nothing particularly wrong with Caitlin's instruction, but I found it jarring: in my experience, supervision was for learning how to think, not being told what to do. And while I didn't imagine I would have any more success than the previous therapist with getting Carmen to come regularly, the last thing I wanted was to begin my relationship with her with the shared assumption that she would miss her sessions. I told Caitlin about one of my former supervisors, who'd said that she never talked about cancellation policies with patients until after they had actually canceled on her. "If I start by talking about cancellations," Dr. Stein had said, "I'm conveying the message that the therapy is not something worth making an effort to show up for. Instead, I start with the idealistic and unspoken notion that the work will be gratifying and that of course the patient will come every single time." Caitlin was unimpressed.

"You'll see," she said. "She's going to stand you up."

"She'll stand me up no matter what I say or don't say," I replied.

"Still, I'll hate to have to say I told you so."

Somehow I doubted that. Just then embarking on what would be a yearlong relationship with Caitlin, I already felt not only completely dismissive of her skills but also utterly defeated. None of this would be good for any of the parties involved and, as I knew in my gut on that first day, least of all for the patient who'd unwittingly landed in the midst of us.

CHAPTER THREE

IF DR. YOUNG WAS TECHNICALLY MY SUPERVISOR AT FOREN-
sics, it soon became clear that this was only technical. She
waved each morning when she walked past me and into her
office, and sometimes if we rode the elevator together, she
would turn to me and ask an oddly timed personal question,
like did I want children. (I did; she did not.) I had long ago,
if with some regret, abandoned my notion that psychologists
would necessarily have good interpersonal skills, and I found
Dr. Young more likable than some. She was quite cheerful
and had given me that good advice about what to do if I got
stopped by the police, which, the more time I spent around
the hapless defendants, the easier it was to imagine as a likely
eventuality. Dr. Wolfe was often around to provide thoughtful answers to my recurring questions about the defendants we
saw, and so rather than request the face-to-face time with Dr.
Young that I was only half sure I was supposed to be having
anyway, I took to following the master's students around like
a lamb. Another day, another 7:30.

One morning and then another, and how quickly they became so similar. Dr. Matthew Laytner, Dr. Pine, Jim Danziger, and I began with Robert Woodhale, who knew who he was but could not quite say where he was. "At Rikers?" he asked, which was not a bad guess given the bars confining us to the courthouse's basement holding cell. "At Bellevue?" he tried again, another good guess because of course he'd been confined there before.

From what I'd seen, Mr. Woodhale was the epitome of competency assessment referrals: twenty-seven years old, a string of arrests that made a neat pairing with his string of psychiatric hospitalizations. He was African American, soft-spoken, dressed in a hospital gown and dirty sweatpants, sneakers without laces, handcuffs. When asked for his Social Security number, he recited what must have been his zip code.

Dr. Laytner—a young, good-looking psychiatrist who was as new to the forensic team as I—explained that though he was a psychiatrist, this talk was not confidential, that rather it was an assessment for the court. "Do you know why?" asked Dr. Laytner, whose careful grooming was cast in especially high relief against this backdrop.

"To avoid me staying in an institution?" Mr. Woodhale asked.

"You were arrested," interjected Jim Danziger, looking up from his highlighter and his magazine. He also had Mr. Woodhale's file in front of him. "Do you know what you were arrested for?" Mr. Woodhale shook his head. "You hit a guy at your group home in the face with a chair," Jim told him. It was not a courtroom thriller.

Dr. Pine listened and took her own notes for the brief report that she or I would need to write later. I had not yet asked to conduct an interview—as the master's students often did—but I had jumped wholeheartedly into writing them up afterward, in three pages or fewer. Dr. Laytner tried to get a coherent social history from Mr. Woodhale. He failed. Mr. Woodhale could not say how he had spent the last year; he was preoccupied with getting his disability check. Then he remembered: "Schizophrenic, I'm schizophrenic. I have a mental illness."

"Do you know what medications you take?" asked Dr. Laytner.

"Geodon," said Mr. Woodhale.

"Do you know what it's for?"

"Schizophrenia."

"Do you hear voices?" asked Dr. Laytner.

"I hear your voice," replied Mr. Woodhale.

"Can you explain to me what your legal situation is now?" asked Dr. Laytner, continuing with the evaluation.

"You tell me that," said Mr. Woodhale. "Explain to me please."

"I need you to try to explain it to me," said Dr. Laytner patiently.

"Hmm, let's see, what's facing me. I'm just waiting until I get out. Two years. Three years. It was hot out. They're homosexuals. They know my name. They're after my money."

Mr. Woodhale was escorted out of the holding cell. Later, Dr. Pine and Dr. Laytner would have no trouble agreeing that this defendant—unclear as he was on whether he had even been arrested—was not fit to stand trial.

The corrections officer returned with our second evaluation of the morning, a Mr. Ramone. "Call me Paulie," said the big-gutted, blustery Italian man in his fifties. His hair was bleached blond with dark roots. He had one black eye. He was wearing a plaid bathrobe and carrying a Bible. Paulie's presence was like a shot of hard liquor, and the mood in the room lightened. Immediately, we all knew he was manic, or using manic defenses—primarily denial and acting out—in order to escape distress and avoid feelings of loss. Most everyone uses manic defenses once in a while, and they can be fairly benign. I was familiar with them firsthand, having spent more than a few afternoons in furies of cleaning and errands when I was fighting a black mood. But on the more pathological end of the spectrum, mania can dislodge rational thought and completely disrupt a life.

Dr. Laytner introduced us all, our smiles now broad, and asked Paulie if he knew why he was there. "To see if I'm sane," Paulie replied, smirking. "You can't build appliances for twenty-nine years and be insane, sir."

"When did you do that to your hair?" asked Dr. Laytner, responding to the jovial mood in the room while also asking an important question about the inmate's history—that is, how long had he been sick enough to make himself look so odd.

"After my wife left," Paulie said proudly. "The girls love it. I get more winks and smiles than I ever did with the gray. You can see why, right, sweetheart?" he asked, turning to me. I smiled wider and nodded.

"What happened to your eye?" Dr. Laytner inquired.

"I'm not a violent person," said Paulie. "I love people. I'm a lover. I was a hippie, sir."

"It says here that you got into a fight with your cell mate," said Jim, reading from the file.

"Without the Klonopin, everything bothers me," explained Paulie. "It seems like everyone wants to fight with me. Once I'm out, the only medication I'll need is my Harley."

Dr. Laytner explained why we were gathered there and

made Paulie aware that our talk was not confidential. He gave him a consent form to sign. "No problem. I've got nothing to hide," he said.

"Do you know what you're accused of?"

He sighed. "I'm getting divorced. I drove my Cadillac through the garage door. But it wasn't my fault. It was an accident."

"Anything else?"

"No. Well, okay, barricading myself in my house. My wife had an order of protection against me. There was a warrant out for my arrest because they said I'd been driving by the house, which was a lie. I was upstate. My cousin will swear to that."

"Why did you barricade yourself in the house?"

"I didn't! I went over there to watch the Giants game. I didn't even know she'd come home and called the police. I went to sleep and woke up to helicopters and SWAT teams. They stormed into my bedroom to get me. My wife will do anything to put me in jail."

"Why does she want to do that?"

"I'm not in her mind, sir. You'll have to ask her that question."

"Well, what is your best guess?"

"She's mentally ill. This is all part of her evil plan."

"Evil plan?"

"I go to the loony bin for the rest of my life, and she gets everything."

"Do you think that plan makes any sense?"

"Any spouse can lock up any other spouse. It's the law. You should know the law before you come to see me, sir."

"How do you plan on handling your conflict with her?"

"See this Bible? God is with me. I'll make sure the newspapers get my side of the story. I'm going to sell my house and move to Barbados. I'll raise German shepherds. I may still love her, but I'll divorce her. It'll make headlines. She'll regret all this then."

Mania in and of itself does not necessarily make a defendant incompetent. But as Dr. Laytner went on with the interview, it would become clear that Paulie's use of denial was behind his refusal to craft a reasonable plan for dealing with the charges against him. "They're going to be dropped," he kept insisting. "You can't be put in jail for breaking into your own house." Dr. Pine and Dr. Laytner would once again agree: not currently fit to stand trial.

Back upstairs the students milled about the small, tidy forensics office. I stood in Dr. Wolfe's vacant cubicle, looking to see how far he'd gotten in the *Times* crossword puzzle and hoping he'd come back from his morning interviews to chat. What I wanted to talk about I had to keep to myself: how frustrated I was feeling in the G Building, by Scott and Caitlin and what little else was going on there as of yet. I needed someone with some authority to validate my discontent and offer me condolence. To tell me I was right. If I could only get it surreptitiously by talking about the crossword puzzle, I would settle for that, but when Dr. Wolfe arrived, I became self-conscious and blushed. He looked at me funny. "Is it hot in here?" he asked.

"I get flushed easily," I explained. It was true, but maybe I also had a schoolgirl crush on him. It was hard, sometimes, to differentiate between all the kinds of longing.

Dr. Wolfe sat down at his desk, and I settled across from him. Apropos of nothing obvious, he began to tell me a story about a job interview he had once sat in on. The male psychologist doing the interview had taken it upon himself to confront the female interviewee with what he supposed was the "fact" that she wanted to sleep with him. The story was tangentially related to earlier discussions Dr. Wolfe and I had had about my theoretical orientation, about the flouting of social convention that he viewed as a point of pride among psychoanalytically oriented clinicians. But why had he associated to that particular story in that particular moment? As happened more and more the longer I was in school, I couldn't stop myself from thinking like a therapist. My training had taught me to pay attention to associations: each new idea is linked to the one that came before it. I imagined Dr. Wolfe believed my blushing a sign that like the interviewee in his story, I was harboring prurient thoughts. Given our age difference, I hoped he would only be flattered, but in moments like those I often felt I'd rather not be privy to the ways of knowing of my field. I was certainly not a mind reader, as strangers I met at parties sometimes seemed to fear, but like a telepath I did have clues to bits of others' private thoughts that a non-psychologist was spared. I guessed that I could never go back to being that, and my chest filled with regret.

When a defendant had the money to make bail, he could walk into the courthouse like a free man and meet with us up on the thirteenth floor. Because people with such abundant resources rarely needed our services, I saw this happen only once. The man was kempt and handsome, in suspenders and a navy blazer with a yellow tie. Despite this sartorial care, there were strings hanging from the bottom of his pants, as if he were waiting to unravel. His name was John Douglass. He'd been arrested for having a loaded gun but no permit. The police found him sitting in his car with it contemplating suicide.

"My wife saw me leave the house and called them because she knew my state of mind," he explained. "I had it for target shooting. I just hadn't ever bothered to renew the license." He referred to his arrest as "the incident."

"I haven't worked since the incident," he told us. He'd been a newspaperman for more than twenty years. He regretted the changes wrought by technology. "I lived for pasteup—the careful cutting, the precision. Now everything's computerized, and it's just a job."

He'd never been hospitalized, but he'd had problems with cocaine for a long time, giving it up only a couple years before with the help of Narcotics Anonymous. "But then I got addicted to painkillers," he said as he began to cry. "I've put my wife through so much. It's been the usual craziness that comes with abuse. Lying. Money problems. I drank four or five quarts of beer and took nine Percocets, and I went out to end my life."

Dr. Wolfe asked if he'd ever thought about suicide before.

"No, just in this past year. I couldn't believe I was capable of this moral and physical decay."

He was sleeping okay. Eating, too. He was planning on returning to work. He was not confused or unable to communicate with his lawyer, but there was concern that the pressures of a trial would drive this still emotionally fragile man back down to a place that was dangerously bleak. It had only been two weeks since the incident.

For the time being, the doctors agreed he was unfit.

In school I had learned that the emotional pull toward the grossest distortion of external reality—psychosis—takes root or doesn't in the first year of life, from some combination of nature and nurture. If what's going on in a baby's environment is too dreadful to accept, or if innate characteristics result in said baby experiencing his world in that way, he may never lay to rest the most frightening concerns of early life, which psychologists think of as engulfment and annihilation. Extremes of environment or biology or some combination of either can impede an infant's ability to accomplish two of the basic emotional tasks of the first year: realizing that he exists as a separate being, and establishing a rudimentary trust in those around him. If there is a relationship in which a baby receives sufficient soothing, and if his brain allows it, these tasks become faits accomplis. If not, a person will go through life vulnerable to the fears that luckier people master early, in times of stress becoming psychotic or dependent upon the primary defenses used by infants to hold himself together.

Psychologists label the earliest defenses "primitive" and mean that in the most literal (read: non-pejorative) sense: developmentally early. The primitive defenses, in contrast to "higher order" ones, reflect qualities associated with a child's preverbal phase of development—lack of understanding of reality, and lack of appreciation of the separateness and constancy of others. The primitive defenses include colloquially familiar ones like denial and projection—when feelings that originate inside the self are misunderstood as coming from others. They also include less familiar ones like introjection, when what is threatening and outside is experienced as if coming from within, and omnipotent control—the fantasy that one controls the external environment with one's mind. The use of each can result in psychotic symptoms. Some of these symptoms, like stilted turns of thought, are subtle enough to escape casual notice. Others are more florid: hallucinations, delusions, acute paranoia, and the like. It was these that were almost always on display at forensics, and seeing them up close for the first time felt valuable, even if I wasn't getting to do any treatment.

Illogical thinking is one artifact of psychosis, and the defendants we saw often had interesting ideas about how they'd become ill. Mr. Ruiz, with his salt-and-pepper hair and the same date of birth as my mother, attributed his confusion to a watermelon seed. "I swallowed it, and I felt it go up into my head," he told us. "It's causing trouble. I feel it there now, and I can no longer think very well. When I was young, my mind was okay, but not now." His crime was trespassing, though by his account his trespass was only into his former home, an abandoned building where he'd squatted for three years before the absent owners insisted he leave. "They turned on me," he said glumly. He'd been homeless much of his life. He wore a sweatshirt tied around his neck like a cape. He would not agree to either take a plea or go to trial, and he kept insisting, "I can't pay these people," meaning his lawyer, though it was repeatedly explained to him that someone else would cover the expense. Mr. Ruiz was not fit to stand trial.

I climbed back upstairs to wait for the next round of interviews and was sitting in the clinic's reception area when Dr. Ruben tore into the office in worked-up excitement. He had done an evaluation of a highly distractible defendant. Accused of robbing people on the subway, a crime the man claimed not to remember, he seemed unable even to follow his evaluators' conversation. Furthermore, he could not understand why he could not simultaneously claim lack of memory of the event *and* that he hadn't been carrying a gun. Dr. Ruben wanted to argue the defendant unfit on the basis of attention deficit disorder. He was an older psychiatrist, educated before attentional disorders were a point of focus, but he'd recently been

reading about them in the *New York Times*. He was asking the
clinic secretary if she could order the paper-and-pencil tests
used to diagnose it when I interjected to tell him that the hospital already likely had them, and also offered to do the testing
myself. I knew that ADD on its own did not cause the level of
inattention Dr. Ruben described, but I thought it could be an
interesting assignment and was ready to do something more
active than sitting in on evaluations, which were never boring
but were starting to feel repetitive nonetheless.

Dr. Young overheard my offer and popped her head out
of her office to endorse it. She agreed that even if our guy had
ADD, it was likely to be the least of his problems given, naturally, his very long history of psychiatric hospitalizations and
arrests. Still, the testing would help fulfill one of my training
requirements (five or six full testing batteries), and it would
satisfy Dr. Ruben's nascent curiosity. It was a win–win. And
so the sporadically homeless, often incarcerated, and chronically mentally ill Grant Carson, as the defendant was named,
became the unlikely subject of an extensive psychological
screening.

Generally, psychologists do two kinds of testing, cognitive
and personality, and I'd done a fair amount of both in graduate
school. Cognitive tests measure IQ and educational achieve-
ment. They're used to diagnose learning disabilities, including ADHD, and to quantify other intellectual abilities, most
often when they seem on the decline, say after a head injury,
or if some kind of dementia is settling in. Personality tests
look at different aspects of a person's cognitive, emotional, and
interpersonal functioning. Some of them involve self-reports,
where the participant answers a series of questions about himself. Others are projective, which means the subject is presented with an ambiguous stimulus like an ink blot and asked

to make meaning of it, offering clues to his emotional preoccupations. Cognitive and personality tests are ideally given in conjunction, as the two areas are inextricably intertwined, our intellect shaped or constrained by our character.

The first time I met with Grant Carson, it was not to administer any test but simply to hear about his life. I went into the basement on my own for the first time, down the very long staircase, and found him sitting, lanky limbed and bent, on the metal bench that lined the back wall of the holding cell. He was staring at the gray cement floor beneath his laceless boots. He did not look up when I introduced myself and explained why I was there, though he did stick out his cuffed hands meekly to shake mine. His long neck craned downward, his eyes hidden in shame, he was the most pitiful being I'd ever seen, like a woodland creature awaiting transformation in a fairy tale. Though he was almost fifty, he looked like a little boy, something in his face and the way he was folded. I sat down at the table in front of him and put down my notebook and pen. "How are you doing today?"

"I'm tired," he said, still looking at the floor. His tone and prosody did nothing to lend credence to the idea that he was a grown man. "I don't sleep much at Rikers."

"How come?" I asked.

"My mother comes to see me in the middle of the night. She sits next to me and we talk. She died of cancer a few years ago, so the only time I get to see her is when she shows up real late."

I nodded and thought. "What do you talk about?"

"About when I was a child. I tell her if she'd loved me, she wouldn't have let my stepfather rape me. She tells me I'm worthless and that I should shut up."

"What's that like for you?"

"She's a real comfort," he said, nodding his head and rocking back and forth.

"How long has she been coming to see you like that?"

"She started when I was in Attica."

Grant Carson went on to describe his life, more than a third of it spent in one type of prison or another. His longest stint had been ten years at Attica Correctional Facility in upstate New York, not too long before our meeting. The charges had always been similar: robberies he could not recall, criminal possession of weapons, drugs. He told me he started using marijuana at age seven, the year after his stepfather began sodomizing him in his closet on an almost daily basis. When he wasn't being raped himself, he could hear the man in the next room with his sister. "I used to see her crying in her room, and I knew."

His stepfather threatened to kill the children's mother if they told, and Grant kept quiet. He began responding to a voice that no one else could hear around age nine, was disruptive in class, and got suspended or expelled multiple times. His family doctor labeled him hyperactive. His stepfather died when Grant was fifteen, but the man continued to haunt him in his dreams, where his appearance was enough to make Grant get up and run in his sleep. He began drinking at eleven and using crack at sixteen and angel dust at twenty. He got what passed for help—that is, antipsychotic medication—for the first time in jail at age twenty-five. He'd never had any kind of talk therapy. During his time away from jail, he'd fathered a child every few years—none of the five now wanted much to do with him. His acting out was like Russian roulette: he'd tried to hang himself dozens of times while at Attica, where the guards would always arrive in time to save him, in time but also much too late.

"Your stepfather never comes to visit like your mother?" I asked.

"No, just in my dreams," he said, shaking his head. "But sometimes Ken comes."

"Ken?"

"He's this white guy." Grant was black. "He's been coming around since I was a kid."

"Do other people know Ken?"

"I'm not really sure," he told me. "When Ken comes, Grant leaves."

I paused at the last part. I'd quickly assumed Ken was just another auditory hallucination, a voice in Grant's head. But if he really experienced himself as leaving upon Ken's arrival, he might be describing an alter, another personality. Dissociative identity disorder (DID), or multiple personalities, is theoretically an outgrowth of early and chronic traumatic experience, so it fit with Grant's history, but there was debate in the field about the disorder's actual existence. Some clinicians identify DID in a large number of their traumatized patients, while others claim it's iatrogenic, or brought on by the treatment itself, by practitioners who want to find it working with patients who are eager to please. I'd taken an entire class on the defense called dissociation, the process that underpins DID. Like all defenses, dissociation is a normal function of the mind, widely experienced, for instance, in the benign form of daydreaming—the daydreamer "leaves" a situation mentally while remaining physically present and physiologically awake. Dissociation also offers protection from overwhelming experiences of terror, as an unbearable event is processed as if not quite happening to the self. Trauma victims commonly describe watching themselves as if from the outside as the very bad thing goes on, and therapy with this population is necessarily focused on integrating the disturbing experiences—making them part of their conscious and continuous life story. Like other defenses, dissociation is only pathological when it becomes a person's go-to way of dealing with even objectively minor life stressors, and this is what theoretically happens in dissociative identity disorder. DID always made sense to me: it just seemed like dissociation reaching its inevitable potential. But I'd never before been seated at a metal table across from someone who had it, and I found it perversely exciting.

"What do you mean Grant leaves?" I asked. There were specific questions designed to clarify whether someone was prone to dissociation, but damn it I couldn't remember them just then.

"Sometimes Ken takes over," he replied.

When I finished my interview with Grant, I went back upstairs and straight to Dr. Wolfe's cubicle—he had been assigned to oversee the case—and he was thoughtful.

"It might explain why he can't remember the robberies," he said. "Or he could be malingering."

It was hard for me to believe that the fragile man who'd sat before me could fake a toothache, let alone anything as elaborate as a white man named Ken, but I agreed the matter warranted more attention. Dr. Wolfe suggested I add a self-report measure that helped flesh out dissociative experiences to the list of tests I'd administer to Grant, and he told me he'd want to speak to Grant himself before the testing was through. We told Dr. Ruben, the psychiatrist who'd made the referral, that I suspected DID, and he expressed faux annoyance: he'd had high hopes that this one might be treated with a quick dose of Ritalin and then sent off to trial. "Multiple personalities!" he exclaimed under his breath and walked off, shaking his head.

The next week Grant was returned to the courthouse twice

to take hour upon hour of tests. Given that our mutual efforts would likely culminate in the conclusion that he, like all the others, was unfit to stand trial, it seemed like overkill, but who was I to say? First thing in the morning, he was waiting for me in the basement holding cell, his head held low. We started with the WAIS—the Wechsler Adult Intelligence Scale. David Wechsler, the American psychologist who developed the test, defined intelligence as "the global capacity of the individual to act purposefully, to think rationally, and to deal effectively with his environment." The test measures verbal and nonverbal abilities, and it's how you arrive at someone's IQ. Some parts of the test involve learning a new skill, and these measure what is called fluid intelligence, while others look at fund of knowledge, or crystallized intelligence. Generally speaking, intelligence is impacted by a lot of things. Like every aspect of being, some of it has to do with innate capacity, and some of it has to do with environment. Grant had only gone as far as the ninth grade, and given all the abuse he was enduring at home, it wasn't likely he was able to focus on what was going on in the classroom, whether or not he had ADHD. As Grant and I moved through the different parts of the test, it was obvious he wasn't doing well. We'd been carrying on for a while when he couldn't define one of the vocabulary words I presented to him, and he looked as if he might break down. I stopped to ask why he thought he was getting so upset.

"I want to do well because then I'll feel happy," he answered, and I couldn't say which I thought was less likely.

After Grant and I had spent two days and many hours engaged in the Rorschach, the Thematic Apperception Test, the Delis-Kaplan Executive Function System, and the Test of Memory Malingering, among others, on yet another morning Dr. Wolfe came down with me to meet Grant and to administer the Multidimensional Inventory of Dissociation (MID), to determine once and for all if our guy had multiple personalities. Grant spoke a little differently of the white man named Ken this time around, and it was hard to say whether he was a hallucination or an alter. The MID wasn't a huge help because while Grant agreed that yes, he had trancelike episodes where he stared off into space and lost awareness of what was going on around him, felt uncertain about who he really was, and relived traumatic events so vividly that he totally lost contact with his surroundings, he didn't always seem to completely comprehend the statements he was endorsing. Dr. Wolfe was not convinced, and I didn't know what to think. With so much trauma in his history and so many symptoms in his present, it was difficult to parse the whole thing out. This was almost always the case with our defendants, though Grant was an extreme example. Dr. Wolfe and I settled on a diagnosis of chronic post-traumatic stress disorder, among others.

Every testing report ends with recommendations, and beyond suggesting that Grant be found unfit to stand trial, ours came down to this: get this guy some serious psychological help. I had never before so vehemently hoped that my recommendations would be implemented, but given that Grant still stood accused of holding up honorable citizens at gunpoint on the subway, and that the justice system had limited resources when it came to mental health care, I doubted he would ever get the therapy he'd need to have any relief. Grant Carson was probably the first person I'd ever met who made me question whether significant relief was always even a possibility. Maybe a person could only take so much. Maybe there was a point of psychological no return.

As one month passed at forensics and then another, I began to be acutely discomfited by the fact that I had yet to actually conduct a fitness-to-stand-trial evaluation. The students were allowed, if never outright encouraged, to do this—to go through the standard interview protocol with a defendant while the doctors looked on. Given that these evaluations were more or less all that went down in the court clinic, I felt conspicuous about my reluctance, my self-appointed status as the wallflower at the orgy. I'd grown up with a critical father. I'd gone on to choose first one and then another career where I could make others the explicit focus of attention—perhaps no one need notice me—but now there was this live audience. At forensics I'd looked on as the master's students led the assessments, and I knew I couldn't do much worse. One particularly shiny-haired girl had giggled most of the way through, to the point where I cringed mightily for the defendant, whose business there was not a laughing matter. In the laid-back court clinic, where responsibility for teaching was after all so diffuse, no one was going to suggest that I do anything. It was all up to me, which made my reticence feel all the more like a personal failure.

Dr. Wolfe walked back to collect a couple students. I had stopped waiting a beat to volunteer to go downstairs to watch, and so I stood up right away. The mood that day was jovial. Dr. Wolfe and Dr. Laytner were excited about this case, a young man who had tried to kill his family with a samurai sword. It had dramatic overtones and a potentially compelling narrative, at least relative to the heavy rotation of disturbers of the peace who so often filled our days.

It was actually starting to feel monotonous, all that craziness I was not there to learn to treat, and so I had decided—with Scott's approval—that I would leave the court clinic for good that week, a month early. All the commuting back and forth midday had proven a disappointing way to spend my time, and also I guessed, having gotten a feel for what profound mental illness looked like, I'd learned as much as I was going to there. One rotation or another had to be cut short by a compulsory month in the psychiatric emergency room anyway. Beginning the next week I would be at the hospital full-time.

From the other interns' experiences—shared in fitful bursts before our seminars and during our weekly intern support group—I understood this would be a mixed bag. My sense that psychologists might be dismissed by the psychiatrists who ruled the G Building had been correct, to the extent that the M.D. in charge of the inpatient unit that Jen, Leora, Zeke, and Alisa had been assigned to had refused to give them patients at all. Instead, this psychiatrist distributed therapy duties among the third-year medical students, who, while they had passed gross anatomy, had likely never as much as taken Psych 101. Scott had tried to intervene to no avail, and our director finally settled on moving the interns to a different unit altogether, but not before we'd all learned a pointed lesson about the dismissive arrogance of psychiatry. Until then it had been for us mostly a myth.

On our trek down the long courthouse staircase, Dr. Wolfe told me Scott had asked him to supervise the women's depression group I had recently begun co-leading in the outpatient clinic. Each of the five forensic psychologists spent one day a week at the hospital proper, so many of them supervised non-forensic goings-on. Dr. Wolfe's news was especially welcome because with forensics coming to a sudden close, I had regretted cutting ties with him, the only psychologist I'd so far found to look up to. It was proving hard, at this institution under siege, to locate someone willing to take on that role. If there was an every-man-for-himself ethos in Behavioral Health that year, I could hardly blame the staff, who from the junior psychologists on up seemed themselves without solid leadership. Still, I felt a lack. I had started co-leading a support group for cancer patients as they waited for their chemo, and my warm but impossibly overstretched oncology group supervisor canceled about half the time. I had signed up for a seminar on family therapy, which included taking on a family case, and my supervisor for that was equal parts helpful and scatterbrained—"I got held up at the bank" was the best he could do after forgetting to show up for what would have been our third-time-rescheduled second meeting. ("At gunpoint?" Jen asked, not altogether kidding, when I repeated his words to her later.) We'd started an interesting psychopharmacology class, but the psychiatrist teaching it only managed to make it once in a while. While Caitlin Downs never canceled a supervision, our time together was so unsatisfying I wished she would. Dr. Wolfe was available *and* knowledgeable about psychology, and after all these weeks seemed fond of me. As small a bright spot as that was in the larger picture of my training, it was sustaining.

Joseph de la Paz sat waiting in the basement holding cell. He was small, in his mid-twenties, and with the by-now-familiar history—his education cut short when his thoughts began to feel scrambled, his sporadic drinking and drug use becoming heavier as his psychotic symptoms intensified. He was obsessed with homosexuality and homicide. Mr. de la Paz traced the origin of his problems to his aunt, with whom he lived. She'd put something in his soup, something she had gotten from a "homosexual" who also happened to be a witch doctor. He feared that people were out to destroy him. He'd purchased the sword at a mall in order to protect himself from his aunt and her gay witch doctor friend and anyone else who might be involved in conspiring against him.

"Why would they want to hurt you?" asked Dr. Laytner.

"Because now women don't respect men," replied Mr. de la Paz.

"But why hurt you in particular?" he followed up.

"Because in America there are a lot of homosexuals," replied Mr. de la Paz.

"But why you?" persisted Dr. Laytner.

"Only God knows," he concluded.

The guard led him out of the cell while we remained. During the interview he had become suspicious of the lawyer Jim Danziger, who he feared might be under the control of the witch doctor. He would not talk to Jim, and so he would be found unfit. As we waited for the next defendant, I gathered my determination and requested to lead the 7:30. Dr. Laytner and Dr. Wolfe said sure. To be polite, I thought, they changed the subject and looked away, allowing me and my nerves some time alone. But my trepidation was for nothing. The guard came in to report the defendant was refusing to see us. The morning was over, I had to go back to the hospital, and telling myself that at least I'd tried, I would not volunteer again.

On my last day at the court clinic, Dr. Young called me into her office for the first time. Because my days at forensics were ending, she needed to formally evaluate me. She had a form for this on her desk, and I could see the Likert scale on which she was supposed to rate me, one through five—five being the best—on various dimensions. She read the first item aloud to me. "'Student was able to incorporate new material effectively.' How do you think you rate on that?" she asked.

"Uh, well, this was all new, and I think I get what these fitness evaluations are all about, so good, I guess," I replied, looking at her questioningly. Did she want me to choose a number?

"Okay, well, let's say we give you a four on that?" She marked it and went on. "'Student applied existing knowledge to new situations.' How about that?"

"I didn't have existing knowledge about forensics when I got here, so I'm not sure that one applies," I said.

"Well, there's no 'NA' choice. It seems like you didn't do that very well, I guess. I'm going to give you a two," she said, making a sympathetic face and then checking the box with her pencil. She presented more statements and waited for my quantitative judgments. When I hesitated to give myself a ringing endorsement on any item, she made a sorry face—not apologetic, more like she regretted my incompetence—and gave me a one or a two. Around question ten, I decided to bring up the fact that maybe someone who knew me better should be filling out the form. She waved away my concerns. "It's not important anyway," she said.

"To you it is unimportant," I wanted to say. "To me it is not."

When this absurdity reached its conclusion, I walked out of Dr. Young's office and shut the door. I realized I probably should have asked for more direct supervision from her weeks before. I would have learned something from it. Dr. Wolfe was standing nearby making copies.

"What's wrong?" he asked. My face always gave me away, but of course it wasn't appropriate to register my complaints about his nominal boss.

"I don't think that internship is going to make me a better therapist" was the best I could come up with, realizing only as I said it that I was actually concerned, given the way things were going, that this was true.

"Maybe not," he said thoughtfully. "But it will make you a better psychologist."

I had been very good at being a graduate student. After my first semester I'd even gotten a letter—bizarre in retrospect because what could have been the point?—informing me that I'd been selected among the best in my class. But it was one thing to be a good doctoral candidate and another altogether to be a good psychologist. My friends who'd gone to law school had all eventually observed that three years in classrooms had taught them about the law but hadn't prepared them to work as lawyers. I'd never thought about the parallel to my own education, though now it seemed so clear. My training was in long-term work with relatively high-functioning people, with the goal of achieving character change. If every patient I encountered on internship could use a really good therapist, given the acute problems they showed up with, a talking cure was never going to be the most immediate concern.

I had arrived in East Flatbush guessing that I would be unwelcome at a hospital, where the first line of defense was always medication, which I could not prescribe. But what was also starting to coalesce was that even if it embraced nonmedical interventions, the hospital had little reason to welcome me. I knew how to think about people, but while I thought this had to be useful beyond the consulting room (in jail cells, say, or on inpatient wards), I couldn't quite say how. Maybe the goal of internship—the whole point—came straight from Dr. Young's form, *student applied existing knowledge to new situations.* I'd loved grad school and had wanted to believe that internship was simply its continuation, but it was not. It wasn't the place to develop the skills I'd long most coveted, but maybe it would make me this other thing. Not a better therapist, but a better psychologist. Once Dr. Wolfe put it that way it felt like a worthwhile aspiration.

CHAPTER FOUR

"SHE'S NEVER IN BEFORE 11:00."

It was 10:15 on the first morning of my new rotation, and having worked up the resolve to move past the screaming sign above the psych ER's staff entrance ("If you don't have a key, you DON'T belong here"), I was now standing outside Dr. Tsyganova's office smack-dab in the middle of the psychiatric emergency room. A middle-aged woman with deep red tight curls addressed me from across the hall as she unlocked her own office door, painted a shade of pink that turned my stomach like riding in the back of a car. I had arrived at 10:00, officially an hour late, but those were the instructions I'd been given by Dr. T., as she was called. I'd leaned for five minutes, and then another five and then another, against the cool wall to the right of T.'s door, watching not much at all go on along the wide, blank corridor lined with matching salmon-hued doors. A handful of patients paced the ceramic-tiled floors of the ER's three halls—laid out like the letter Y—in various states of undress and morning listlessness. If I'd anticipated chaos, the quiet also felt right. Outside it was daylight, and psychiatric emergencies seemed as if they should take place after dark, like other horror movie tropes. The still air smelled of urine and dust, and I concentrated on breathing through my mouth, knowing I couldn't maintain that for the whole of my month there.

"You're the new intern?" the redheaded woman asked. I nodded and didn't ask what gave me away. She invited me into her office to wait for her dilatory colleague. "She's always late," she told me. "I'm the other ER psychologist—Dr. Brink. You can stay with me until Dr. T. gets here." She looked tough, like a smoker and someone you might call a dame or a broad.

We entered her small, bare office, and I sat down on a plastic chair next to a metal desk strewn with files. The walls, off-white and cinder block, were the most ornate aspect of the room. She turned on the lights, but only one of the fluorescent ceiling bulbs stayed lit, the other flickering briefly and then going dark. "It's nicer like that," I observed.

"Not if you're paranoid," she said, picking up her phone to ring maintenance.

When she finished her call, she took a stack of papers from a pile and began scanning them. "New patient, came in last night, brought in by Mom. She'd been throwing up before she arrived and was complaining of stomach pains. When anyone comes in with acute medical problems, they're seen by a physician before they're admitted." She paused for a moment and then added, "Hopefully."

She went back to her scanning. "She was diagnosed with schizophrenia at her last hospital, but the M.D. who saw her last night thought bipolar." She shrugged. Psychiatric diagnosis was famously inconsistent. "I'm going to get her. You can watch me do the interview," Dr. Brink said. She got up and made a move to leave but then turned to me abruptly. "Don't open the door for anyone."

As she left, I glanced into the hallway. Still no sign, at 10:30, of Dr. T.

Dr. Brink brought the patient in. She was a small black woman, wearing dark jeans and a tight black T-shirt. The eyeholes on her sneakers were shiny and vacant. She was my age. Her mother had found her the night before, yelling and with her head in the toilet bowl. I sat silent as Dr. Brink asked her questions about her life. She'd been a paralegal and married. Now she was neither, just in and out of hospitals, on and off medications. She lived with her mother and rarely went out. She was lonely. Her mother came in to answer more questions, and the older woman's upset for her daughter made me want to cry from deep. We'd been together for half an hour or so when there was a knock on the door and Dr. Brink got up and opened it a smidge. Dr. T., dark haired and fiftyish, was standing on the other side looking irritated. "Come on," she said to me, her voice shrill through the crack, spinning on the hem of her slacks without acknowledging her colleague. It was now well after 11:00. Dr. Brink opened the door wider and called after her: "I don't want anyone to accuse me of stealing an intern!" I followed my new supervisor across the hall.

"You don't work for Dr. Brink," Dr. T. said as we sat down at yet another very old desk in an office as spare as her colleague's. From what I'd seen, no one at Kings County did much to decorate, as if they might decide to flee on short notice and couldn't risk leaving anything behind. Or maybe the larger squalor of the hospital just dampened all enthusiasm for aesthetics. In our first weeks, the interns had made plans to improve our own office, as well as the rooms we were to use in the ramshackle outpatient clinic, but we'd so far failed to keep our promises to each other: no posters had been tacked to the walls, no curtains had been hung.

T. harrumphed and straightened some papers. Scott had prepped me for my month with her by suggesting that he found her disagreeable, which made me feel a delectable kinship with her right off the bat despite her apparent commitment to sparing all pleasantries. She and I had known each other, though not well, for a couple of months. She'd been teaching what was so far the interns' favorite seminar, on inpatient intake. Every Friday since late July we'd been filing down to CPEP—the official name for the G Building's ER, the Comprehensive Psychiatric Emergency Program—to watch her interview a person fresh to the place. With patients she was often gentle, but when she spoke to anyone else, she almost always sounded as if she were scolding them.

"You weren't here yet. Dr. Brink was just trying to be helpful," I said.

"I doubt that," said T. "Anyway, I will give you the key to my office so you have somewhere to put your things when you arrive before me. You usually come in at nine, right?" I nodded. She reached into her bag. "I wasn't supposed to make a copy, so don't tell anyone you have this," she instructed. There were so many secrets and allegiances to track.

Dr. T. went on to give me a brisk primer in how things worked in the psych ER. Patients could arrive in two ways. About half walked in on their own asking for evaluation or admission. Not everyone who requested admission was granted it, but when they were deemed suitable, they could sign the papers for a voluntary stay. The others were brought involuntarily by police or paramedics dispatched by concerned third parties. Involuntary admissions required an applicant, usually a family member or hospital administrator, and then the signatures of two physicians: medical doctors of any variety, but not psychologists. At this I raised my eyebrows, to which T. gave a hurried shrug. She had little time to mind such territorial disregard for her expertise.

"My job here, and the one you will be helping me with, is running the EOB, which stands for Extended Observation Bed unit. It's for patients who aren't well enough to leave right away, but who aren't necessarily sick enough to be admitted upstairs to an inpatient unit. We admit people to EOB when we believe they are likely to become stable within seventy-two hours. At the end of seventy-two hours they 'time out,' which means they're either discharged or sent upstairs. Did you notice the two rooms at the end of this hallway? There are three EOB beds in each. One room is for women, the other for men.

"I see each of the EOB patients every day to talk to them and check on their progress. You will be running a group first thing every morning for the six patients. It's as much a community meeting as a therapy group. The idea is that EOB is milieu treatment, which means the environment itself is therapeutic. The ER can be a difficult place to be. You're held here, and there's no one to ask questions of. The psychiatrist comes by for a minute, a nurse, maybe a social worker. Lots of tension builds up. The group is really important because it's where patients can get information and have a chance to voice what it's like to be here. Your job is to help them think about why they're here and how they can use this environment positively."

Dr. T. explained some particulars of the group and added that once it wrapped up each day, I would generally spend the rest of my morning in the ER seeing patients with her. She suggested I walk around and get acclimated. "Make sure to trust your instincts out there," she said, gesturing toward the hallway. "Rely on your feelings. If a patient is making you anxious, walk away. Move slowly, make eye contact, speak soothingly—'Come, let's get some juice' or 'Let's go talk to the nurse.' And get friendly with the staff. You never know when you're going to need someone's help."

I was dismissed. I left T.'s office. The halls became livelier as the morning wore on and the manic energy worked its magic, and I relaxed a little more. There were handfuls of patients up and about, some sitting in the dayroom's plastic chairs staring at the television, others pacing the hallways or leaning against walls. Two police meandered in with a dirty man in handcuffs between them (I would learn to term him "poorly groomed") and made their way to the nursing station to check him in. A couple of flies buzzed about—I recognized them from our ER seminars. A fat black woman in a red bra and a full-length black skirt was walking in circles at the hub of the corridors chanting "Jesus is coming, in Jesus's name" over and over and then over again. I stayed as long as I could bear and then let myself out with my skeleton key. As I reentered the main lobby of G and felt myself exhale fully for the first time that morning, I realized how relieved I was to be leaving the locked ward and just how ambivalent I felt about returning the next day.

- - - - - - - - -

But it was an ambivalence tinged with delight. I both did not want to be in CPEP and would not have traded it for any rotation in the world. If I could only absorb its lessons without having to spend any time there, in the near stench. Twenty-one hours later, I unlocked the door and passed the guard stationed inside. I walked down the quiet hall to T.'s office and let myself in, putting down my things. Her computer was still on, and the garbage was filled with grease-stained food wrappers left by the psychiatry residents on duty the night before. I wondered what went on in the psych ER in the middle of the night. I was sure it was horrible because mornings had a calm-after-the-storm feel. I half wished psychologists were deemed necessary during off-hours. That we weren't seemed just one more endorsement of psychiatry's primacy, of its greater import.

I checked my e-mail to delay my next task, which was to gather the EOB patients for my first group. I'd lamented that the court clinic required so little of me, and I was eager to see more action here, but it felt taxing in its unfamiliarity, and it was October but still so damn hot. At 9:30, I forced myself to close T.'s Web browser and went back into the hallway. Patients were scattered about, eating breakfasts of cold cereal and hard-boiled eggs and bananas off sturdy plastic trays that made me think of my college cafeteria and sledding after the first snowfall, and I felt nostalgia for that languorous time when I might still have chosen any profession in the world.

I cajoled myself into the hallway, and as per Dr. T.'s instructions I walked the short distance to the nursing station at the hub of the Y-shaped space to get the census, the master list of patients who'd been admitted to CPEP. It would say "EOB" next to the names of the six patients registered to T.'s little unit. I knocked and was let in by a nurse's aide. I introduced myself to the head nurse, Miss Higgins, who looked far too busy with a stack of charts and the patients lined up at her window to bother with me. "I'm the new psychology intern," I began. If ever I'd hated a sentence . . . "I need to get the census."

"Ask Rhoda," she directed, glancing my way and then

turning to holler back at the patient yelling at her through the nursing station's window, which was like a ticket seller's at a movie theater, but with thicker, bulletproof glass.

I didn't know Rhoda, and the nurse's aide who'd opened the door for me just shook her head when I looked at her questioningly. I went back into the hallway. One of the psych techs was leaning against the wall. He was young and a little burly, which was par for the course for psychiatric technicians, who as far as I could tell were like the man Fridays of the ER. "Do you know Rhoda?" I asked.

"She's one of the social workers here. Short dark hair," he said. "I think she went outside for a cigarette. What do you need?"

"A census," I told him.

"Hang on," he said. He let himself into the nursing station with his key and came out with a sheet of paper. He handed it to me. "Last night's. But you're working with Dr. T., right? No one was admitted to the EOB since then. This should do." I thanked him and then thought to introduce myself. Though I couldn't imagine any staff member particularly wanting to bother with an intern, T.'s pointed instruction replayed in my head: I was supposed to make friends. I told the tech my name and stuck out my hand to shake his. "Kelvin," he said in response, smiling. "Let me know if you need help finding anybody."

I looked at the list. Only three patients seemed to be registered in the EOB, all men. Dr. T. had said there would be six, but had she meant six max? I walked back down the hall, past T.'s office and into the farthest EOB room, the one for women. Like the rest of the ER, it had a cold concrete floor and frosted windows that couldn't be seen out or smashed. Two patients were inside eating their breakfasts, sitting on vinyl mattresses that had been set into low, wooden platform beds built into the floor. Maybe the females had been accidentally left off the list? "Good morning. Are you EOB patients?" I asked. I felt too harried and sounded it. They stared at me blankly, but I wasn't sure that this ruled them out. Did EOB patients know they were EOB patients? It probably wasn't the first thing on their minds.

"I was sexually harassed at Woodhull!" one hollered at me, putting aside her tray. She was hefty, wearing a gray mini-dress and a cropped denim jacket. Both were a few sizes too small on her. Her words poured out like her flesh where it met the bands of her clothing. "I'm filing charges. I need a lawyer. Are you a lawyer? I was minding my own business. I filed a police report. That's a stack of papers that are read by the police. I am going to launch a lawsuit. A suit is worn by a lawyer, but that is not the same as a lawsuit."

The other woman was dressed in a hospital gown and also seemed to want my attention. She broke in, speaking in slow motion or as if she were underwater. "Excuse me, miss? I'm ready to leave. Can you sign my discharge papers? There's nothing wrong with me." The first woman looked at her with exasperation.

"Excuse me, but I was talking to the lady, putting together words, phrases, sentences, but not the kind they give out in court," said gray dress.

"I'm sorry, but I can't help either of you." This was true, but it sounded so wrong. I tried to come up with something more therapeutic. "Someone else will help you soon. I have to go find the patients on my list," I explained, holding up the census. They looked at me as if I were crazy, and I reinforced that idea by suggesting they have a nice day.

In the men's EOB room next door—identical down to its white peeling paint—I discovered two more patients. One was lying on a vinyl mattress, wrapped from head to toe in a gray flannel blanket. The other was asleep on the hard floor, despite the two empty beds. I saw Kelvin in the hallway and motioned him over. He smiled and walked toward me. I appreciated his good humor. "Should I wake them?" I asked. He approached the man on the floor and nudged him gently with his sneaker.

"You don't ever want to bend over a patient here to wake him up," he explained as he nudged. "You can't be sure what shape he's in. If he's psychotic, or even just startled, he might lash out in response. You don't need to get punched in the face, and he doesn't need to suffer the consequences of hitting you." I nodded. The patient just grumbled and rolled over, his arm slung to his side. Kelvin bent down, keeping as much distance as he could, and read the patient's plastic admission bracelet. He recited the name to me: not on my list. Apparently, anyone could wander into the EOB rooms to get some rest.

Kelvin walked over to the man in the bed. He nudged him as well, with his hand this time, still keeping his distance. The patient pulled the blanket off his face to look at us. I explained who I was and asked his name. Bingo. On the list. "We're going to have a group in the dayroom in a few minutes. Would you like to join us?" I asked. He returned the blanket to his face. It hadn't occurred to me that a patient might refuse, and so I had not asked Dr. T. if group was mandatory. Even if it was, I couldn't imagine how I would enforce attendance. I thanked Kelvin and went to explore the rest of the ER. One down, two to go.

With an aide's help, I found my second patient, an old and sickly looking man, standing in the doorway of the bathroom in his pajamas with urine running down one leg. "I'm going to have to get him cleaned up. Can you talk to him later?" asked the aide. I was still not breathing through my nose but knew instinctively that he stank worse than even the room around him. I wasn't supposed to feel this way—and there was the rub. The first lesson of graduate school in clinical psychology is that "supposed to feel" is a distinctly un-clinical concept, and what you *actually* feel provides important information about a patient's interpersonal world. But I wanted nothing to do with this man. ("Neither did his mother," said the voice of one of my professors in my head.)

"Please," I said, motioning the aide forward. She led him off, holding his arm.

I called my third patient's name out in the small, bleak waiting area at the farthest point from the EOB rooms. No one responded. I walked back to the center of the Y and found a nicer, air-conditioned room with five vinyl reclining chairs next to the nursing station. There was a man sprawled on each chair. I spoke my patient's name once again. This time someone responded. "That's me," he said, opening his eyes. He was dressed and clean enough. I approached him.

"I'm Darcy," I said. "I work in the Extended Observation Bed unit, which you've been admitted to."

He nodded. "I know. Been here before."

"Normally, there's a morning group for EOB patients to help get you oriented, but this morning it'll just be you and I," I said, making the decision not to have a proper group, as if it were not a choice made for me. "Do you have any questions?" I asked. He did not.

I explained that he would be in EOB for a maximum of seventy-two hours and that Dr. T. and I would be speaking with him later to see how he was doing. He seemed content and thanked me for the information. "Just one question," I said to him. "Why are you sleeping in here when you have a bed down the hall?"

He pointed toward a small window air-conditioning unit. "The AC," he said. "It's cooler in here."

It was 10:15 by the time I let myself back into Dr. T.'s office to wait for her. It had taken me forty-five minutes simply to locate three patients and not have a group. "You'll do better tomorrow," Dr. T. assured me when she came in at 11:00 and I told her about my morning.

"Was the census right? Are there only three patients today?" I asked.

"Yes, unfortunately," she said. "I have to talk to admissions. We get a thousand dollars from the state for each bed, but only when they're filled. Sometimes the psychiatry residents forget about us, admit people right upstairs, where there are rarely enough beds. If they can't be transferred to another hospital, which most of them can't be, because they don't have insurance, they end up sitting around the ER for several days waiting for a bed to open up, while they could be in EOB actually getting treatment."

"And what if someone doesn't want to come to group? What do I do?" I asked, telling her about the man in the blanket.

"Once in a while, if someone is new to a medication, he might be too tired to come, but we can't know how a patient's doing if he's in bed all day. Group is a critical part of this experience. You need to be getting across the point that treatment is not just sleeping. We expect them to function here.

"Also, you have to think about the way you say things.

Don't ask 'Would you like to come to group?' But rather 'Get up. It's time for group now.' My son is grown, but when I was learning to do all of this, he was in preschool. I learned how to be good with the patients by watching his preschool teachers. Structure is the trick, with little kids and with psychotic patients. The more things escalate, the tighter the structure you need. But always empathic," she concluded. "So let's go talk to the man in the blanket—Mr. Bonture." She had his chart on her desk and glanced at the admission note before we left her office.

Mr. Bonture was right where I'd left him, asleep, or at least wrapped head to toe in his blanket despite the heat. "Wake up, Mr. Bonture," directed T., standing near but not within arm's reach of the bed. "Mr. Bonture, sit up please," she said. He peered up from his blanket, unwrapped it, and sat up. "Good morning," she said.

"Morning," he replied, groggily. He was wearing a hospital gown.

"How are you doing today?" she asked in a tone one might use with a small child.

"I want to sleep," he said, still groggy.

"This is not a hotel," she said firmly, her voice still up a pitch. "You have to get out of bed and get dressed. You'll feel more awake then. You'll get some food."

"Okay," he said, but turned away from us, lying back down, pulling the blanket only up to his chin this time.

"Have you gotten your medicine today?"

"No," he said, back still turned.

She sighed and explained to me that the hospital's computer program for drugs was not all that efficient. "The private hospitals have a much better one. It costs a million dollars.

We probably lose more than that each year because ours is so subpar."

She turned back to Mr. Bonture. "I want to see you dressed and in my office in half an hour," T. said.

"Okay," he replied.

I followed Dr. T. back into her office, relieved because I figured that she hadn't had much more luck with him than I had. I didn't want to look bad, or at least not any worse.

She continued our lesson. "The ER is not like long-term therapy. In long-term therapy you work with a wide-angle lens. Here we use a telescopic lens. We only talk about the most immediate issues."

She opened Mr. Bonture's chart and showed me the admission note. He lived in a group home for the mentally ill and had been brought to the ER after threatening to kill his roommate. "We'll call his caseworker at some point and ask if he has any history of violence. The note doesn't mention any, but we always need to confirm with collateral sources. When we talk to Mr. Bonture, we'll ask him, 'Do you want to kill your roommate? Do you want to kill yourself?'

"I don't care about his words really. I want to see his emotional reactions. Anyone can tell us they're not homicidal. But is he guarded when he responds? Is he sincere? Affect is such a rich language. To be of use here, you need to learn to read it perfectly. You want to know how deep the psychosis goes. How bad is it. Lean on the sore spot and see how the patient reacts. Become progressively more challenging. You want to see how he responds while he's in here—in this safe environment. You'll see when we interview him."

When Mr. Bonture was up and dressed, he knocked on the door of T.'s office. He was still a little groggy but said he wanted to sit down and talk. He'd been to G-ER before and was presumably well enough to know that release required some cooperation. This was a good sign.

"Are you feeling a little better?" T. asked.

"Yes, a little better."

"Less angry?"

"I'm not angry," he said, shaking his head.

"What happened with your roommate?"

"He disrespected me. He insulted me."

"So what did you do?"

"I told him not to disrespect me."

"What else?" she asked.

"I threatened him." He was sheepish now.

"Threatened what?"

"To kill him. I didn't mean it, ma'am. It was just that he insulted me."

"You can't go around threatening everyone who insults you. What was your plan?"

"I hoped to hurt him," he said emphatically.

"Do you have a weapon?"

He nodded. "My fists," he said. "I'm a boxer."

"You don't look very strong." It was true. He did not.

"I am, ma'am. He's strong, too, though. It would've been a fair fight."

"People on the streets of the city can be insulting. Do you plan to go around beating up everyone who insults you?"

"No, ma'am." Mr. Bonture sounded sincere.

"What are your other options?"

"I'll ignore them. I'm better than that."

When he left, Dr. T. asked if I understood the point of the brief interview.

"You pressed the issue, saw how he reacted. You questioned his judgment and also insulted him, saying he didn't look strong," I said.

She nodded. "The 'insult' was sincere. It was what I was thinking. It's important that you are honest here all of the time. Patients sense when you're disingenuous." She went on, "Maybe he just needed to cool off. His insight and judgment certainly seem to have gotten a little better. I'll talk to the psychiatrist about adjusting his medication. We'll keep him another night and make sure he still looks okay tomorrow. You'll see how he does in group."

Upon arrival on the third day at my new rotation, Dr. T.'s words from the previous morning replayed in my head like a strophic melody. "You'll do better tomorrow." I tried not to dwell on the fact that doing better simply meant successfully gathering a small handful of confused people into one room. To think about the six years I'd spent in graduate school to arrive at this moment was self-defeating. *I was becoming a better psychologist.*

I put my things down in T.'s room and found Rhoda in the office she shared with another of the social workers. I introduced myself and asked for the census. She gave it to me. She was compact, with short hair and a square jaw. She wore jeans and a flannel shirt. She told me that she worked with EOB patients, too, mostly on discharge planning. It seemed no one left CPEP without a post–emergency treatment plan. "I'm sure I'll be seeing you around," she said as I left to gather my patients.

There were five patients on the EOB census, including Mr. Bonture and the man from yesterday who'd needed cleaning off. The EOB rooms were empty, so I headed straight back to the hallway with the nursing station. Patients were lined up in front of a room opposite, from which nurses dispensed pills into tiny paper cups, watching their charges down them with small servings of juice. I called the name of the first woman on my list. "She's with me," one of the nurses told me, looking up from taking a patient's blood pressure. "Right here, but she's deaf. Do you sign?"

"No," I told her. My deficiencies were apparently endless.

I called the names of the two other new patients. One young man responded. He was maybe twenty-one and handsome, with taut but not oversized muscles and in a clean T-shirt and jeans. Relieved because he looked like someone I might encounter outside the psych ER, I explained who I was and told him I'd like to take him down to the group room. He was lucid and agreed, and we walked around the corner and down the hall to the dayroom, across from the EOB beds. The dayroom was lined with plastic chairs attached to one another, and there was a round table in the center. The sickly old man, Mr. Younger, sat in the room eating his breakfast. He was clean today, but pieces of muffin fell from between his few teeth as he ate, the crumbs emerging from his too-thin face like maggots from a corpse. The flies buzzed around. The sun shone in too brightly for comfort. I asked Mr. Younger and the handsome man, Mr. Payne, to stay there while I located the other two. A third woman, not on the EOB list, was sitting at the table. "I don't belong here," she announced to me. "I'm Jewish!" She was the first white patient I'd seen in the ER in three days.

I left the dayroom and went back into the hallway. Uncertain how long the two men I'd corralled would wait, I made haste to find the other two patients, keeping my eye on the dayroom door in case anyone decided to leave. Mr. Bonture was outside T.'s office. "Remember me?" I asked. He nodded. "I'd like you to go to the dayroom to participate in a group." I waved him down the hallway, watching as he headed for his destination while I walked the other way. So close now, I got past my self-consciousness and began calling the name of my fourth and final EOB member, Martina, as I walked. She appeared in front of me groggy and in a hospital gown and rubber-soled socks. Triumphant, I invited her to come with me to the dayroom. When we arrived, the other three were still there, as well as the Jewish woman who didn't belong. I felt some relief in my accomplishment, but then I realized the television was on, which meant my task was not complete. Dr. T. had said the boxy set needed to be quieted for group and turning it off required unlocking the mounted plastic case in which it sat, which meant getting the key to the case from an office down the hall. "I'll be right back!" I said.

"Television key?" I asked unceremoniously, poking my head into a room that Dr. T. had pointed out the day before. Someone handed me a key on a long wooden stick. I grabbed it like a relay racer and was back in the group room within seconds, but even standing on a chair, I could not quite reach the lock. The patients sat waiting. It occurred to me to ask the handsome young man for help, but I thought that if he fell off the chair and was hurt, I would be responsible. Instead, I pulled the table over and climbed onto it in my platform heels. The key did not fit easily into the lock, but I jimmied it until it opened, pushing the power button on the set with a flourish. The room went quiet. My patients looked unimpressed. I climbed off the table.

I introduced myself again and explained to my four charges plus the Jewish woman that this morning's group would be a chance for EOB patients to get oriented and ask any questions they might have. The Jewish woman got up and left. Martina had fallen asleep, her head nodding to one side, her hospital gown falling half-open to display dark stretch marks on her breasts.

"I'd like everyone to introduce themselves and tell the group why you're here," I said. I remembered a truism passed down from a supervisor in grad school: a group is only as strong as its highest-functioning member. I turned to the young, good-looking man and asked him to start.

"I'm Glover Payne. I got upset with my girlfriend and took some pills." He frowned and then nodded at me.

I turned toward Mr. Younger, who was sitting across the small room from me, masticated food still coming out from between his teeth. He did not respond. "Mr. Younger?" I asked. Nothing. I continued around the room. "Mr. Bonture?" I asked.

"When am I going to go home?" he wanted to know.

"I'm not sure. Yesterday, Dr. T. thought you were doing okay. Maybe today?"

Glover Payne spoke again. "How about me?"

"I'm sorry, but I don't know. This isn't a discharge group." I looked at the woman in the hospital gown, hoping she could introduce herself and change the subject. She dozed. I didn't have it in me to wake her.

"Well, can you tell me when the discharge group takes place? I'd like to go to that one," said Glover.

"There is no discharge group," I said, though I was uncertain. "There's only this one. You'll have a chance to talk about discharge later today with Dr. T. Mr. Bonture, Glover told us why he's here. Can you let him know how you ended up here?"

"My social worker brought me," he said.

Glover nodded again. They both looked at me. I wanted

to know more about Glover and his girlfriend and the pills but wasn't sure if this group was too public a setting for such questions. "Are you both getting everything you need?" I asked them. If I couldn't quite be a psychologist, at least I could be a good hostess.

"The food's not too good. I'm going to go for a nice meal when I leave," said Glover.

"I might be leaving today," Mr. Bonture told him.

"So who was it you said we should talk to about getting discharged?" Glover wanted to know.

"Dr. T. will be here later. She'll be able to tell you more." I might as well have been wearing a sign that said "Useless," but anyway there was nothing to be done about it. "Dr. T. and I will be talking to you all one-on-one later," I told them, ending our meeting.

When T. arrived, she picked Mr. Younger and his muffin as her first teaching point. "Doing outpatient therapy is passive. Working in the ER is active. Tell him to wipe his mouth. It's very primitive to have food all over. When adults need to be told to wipe off their faces, they're infantile, no ego boundaries. It's not polite to tell a man to wipe his mouth, but we're providing structure, not politeness. To get along in the world, he needs to know how to take care of his body, so part of our job is to help him be more aware. One of the ways we'll know he's getting better is when we don't have to tell him anymore. Who do you want to see first?"

I told her about Glover and his overdose attempt. "Mood disorder or thought disorder?" she asked. It was the same question she'd been posing to the interns each week in the seminar she taught us. Different from the diagnostic paradigm I'd learned in school (developmental level; character organization), the idea here was that you narrowed it down to mood or thought disorder based on a patient's observable behaviors and reported experiences and then tried to isolate which mood or thought disorder it might be per the *DSM*'s checklists of symptoms and their durations. I'd come to understand, in our ER seminars, that a *DSM* mood disorder diagnosis supposed that depression or mania or both were the patient's primary and debilitating problems, while a thought disorder implied that it was psychosis, schizophrenia being the most serious and organic of these, and with the poorest prognosis.

These were the categories of symptoms most typically addressed in the ER, but there was also a third *DSM* category: personality disorder. Glover had become desperate after a threat of abandonment, which I thought put him in this latter group. Thought disorder, mood disorder, personality disorder: they weren't mutually exclusive. Most of the patients we saw likely had personality problems (or rigid and unhealthy patterns of thought and behavior) along with their psychoses and bipolar depressions, but these were never quite addressed in CPEP, sort of like how you wouldn't immediately treat a patient's osteoporosis if he came to a medical ER with a broken arm.

Dr. T. nodded when I told her my ideas and sent me to the nursing station to get Glover's chart. On my way, a young, slim guy in a blazer and pompadour motioned me toward him. I went over. He came close enough to whisper. "I've got a controlled substance," he said, flashing a prescription pill bottle in his right hand.

I became giddy with the opportunity to think quickly. "Can I have it?" I asked.

"No," he replied, dropping the bottle back into his pocket.

I looked around. Kelvin was nearby. I got his attention

and pointed at the patient. "Kelvin," I said, keeping my voice calm. "He's got a controlled substance."

The tech was taller and broader than the patient, who gave the pills to Kelvin without a fuss, muttering something about Adderall. Feeling heroic, I continued toward the nursing station. I retrieved the chart and went back to T.'s office. I wanted to tell her what I'd accomplished, but I couldn't find the words to give my feat its due. I stayed quiet but must have been swollen with pride. Dr. T. took the chart from me and opened it, reading. ER glory was short-lived.

She shared information about Glover with me as she scanned. "He took fourteen Tylenol and then called his girlfriend and told her what he'd done. She showed up four hours later"—at this she furrowed her brow—"and brought him to the medical ER, where they treated him and discharged him to us. What do we want to know when we bring him in?"

"More detail about what set him off. What exactly happened leading up to the attempt. What did he think was going to happen after the fight? Does arguing always upset him? Has he done this before? Does he have mood symptoms like poor sleep or appetite?"

T. nodded. "What else?"

"Is he still suicidal? Had he been feeling for some time that he wanted to die, or was this impulsive? What made him call for help?"

"Good," she said. "You're thinking about mood and personality disorders, and you remembered the telescopic lens. I'll go get him."

When Dr. T. returned, she had both Glover and his girlfriend in tow. The girlfriend did not look happy to be there. "Chandra was here to visit, so I thought we'd do a couple's session," Dr. T. explained, introducing me. The office was only big enough for three chairs. I gave mine up and perched on the edge of the old metal desk.

The room fell silent. "This is a difficult time for you two," said T.

Chandra glanced at Glover angrily and then back at Dr. T. "There is no 'us two' anymore. We broke up a week ago."

"I see," said T., addressing Glover now. "You did this because you couldn't bear to have her leave you." His shoulders slumped.

Chandra continued. "I don't care what he does. I've had enough. We've been together a year, and he's still sleeping with other girls."

Glover broke in, trying to take her hand. "But, baby . . ."

Chandra pulled her hand away. "There's no more 'But, baby.'" She was visibly shaken, teary.

Glover began to speak. "I love her," he told us. "I don't care about those other girls. I only want her. I took the pills because I got so scared about being without her. And then I call her and she doesn't even show up for hours."

"She was angry," said T.

"It's not my job to take care of you!" Chandra replied, starting to cry. "What am I supposed to do now? Be with him or he kills himself?"

"What about trying to understand him better? Why does he fool around with other girls if he loves you? With understanding can sometimes come change—and forgiveness," T. said.

She turned to address Glover. "Tell me about growing up."

"It was good."

"Who raised you?"

"My dad mostly."

"That's unusual."

"My mom was in and out. They were never together. She moved around a lot. When she was in New York, I saw her sometimes."

"That's sad."

Glover shrugged. T. turned to Chandra.

"There's a little boy in him still longing for Mommy. But once he has her, it's terrifying to be so invested in one person, one person who's always abandoning him. So he needs to shore up his resources, find other mommies in case the important one leaves. This is what he's struggling with. It fuels the cheating. The more he starts to feel dependent on you, the more he needs to do it."

"And so I'm supposed to put up with that just because he didn't have a mother?" Chandra seemed angry at the suggestion.

"No," said T. "But if he's serious about being with you, he can really commit to therapy and start looking at those old feelings. Eventually, he won't need the other women in order to quell his anxiety."

Glover tried to take Chandra's hand again. She pulled it away, crying. "I don't know," she said.

"It's just a thought," said Dr. T. "You two need some time alone. We'll stop for today."

"Are you letting me go home?" asked Glover.

"No. Maybe tomorrow. You and I have more talking to do."

Glover and Chandra left T.'s office. She said to me, "What is the real meaning of choice? Does Glover choose to cheat? Yes, sure, but it's also a behavior that's overdetermined—a lot of factors influence it. Most of our big decisions are overdetermined. Take my choice to work here. I've been here almost twenty years. I grew up in a traumatized household. My parents were raised on the Russian front. They saw family members killed in front of them. In my home it always felt chaotic, like we were waiting for something dire to happen. So this crazy place feels familiar to me, comfortable.

"The way we work with patients, we *are* constantly juggling dire situations. The ER is not an outpatient clinic. There you have the luxury of time. Here you do not. There you let the patient set the pace. Here you are direct and provocative. I love working with cases like Glover's. A patient who's not psychotic comes in at a point of crisis in his life. His defenses are down because this just happened. You can really get in there and help him explore his raw spots—same for Chandra. There's just a brief window while they're vulnerable. I want her to see the damaged child inside Glover. His behavior isn't just dumb; it's motivated by who he was."

"I don't know, Dr. T., she just seemed finished," I said.

"But she was crying."

As I left T.'s office to go about my afternoon, I glimpsed Chandra and Glover down the hall holding on to each other as if for dear life.

- - - - - - - - -

When Glover timed out, his cousin came to take him home. T. told me that he had asked Chandra to pick him up but she declined. The cousin, only a little bit older than our patient, was understandably nervous. "What if he tries to kill himself again?" he asked Dr. T.

"You can keep an eye on him, ask how he's doing, but mostly it's out of your hands," she said, always pragmatic. At T.'s suggestion, I had helped Glover set up an appointment with me at the outpatient clinic for the following week.

Apparently, if he didn't see an intern, he'd be assigned to one of the staff psychologists there, and each staff psychologist had 150 patients in her caseload. T. had tried to instill in Glover the value of understanding himself better, even now—especially now—that the crisis had passed. She told me, once he had gone, that she doubted I'd ever see him again. "But I planted the seed," she said. "Maybe after the next girlfriend leaves him, and he starts feeling desperate again."

T. and I were settling in to discuss the morning's group when Dr. Amony, the debonair Haitian head of CPEP, swept into her office. He needed her immediately. He began to tell a story that sounded like the opening line of a joke. *Lady calls 911 to get a squirrel out of her apartment.* When 911 had failed to materialize some hours later, the lady called back. "How do I get you here?" she asked them. "Do I have to say I want to kill myself? Fine! I want to kill myself!" The police arrived quickly. They brought the lady to CPEP, leaving the squirrel behind to have its way in her pantry.

"We've got to see her and get her out of here," Dr. Amony told Dr. T., making it clear he feared litigation if she wasn't quickly evaluated and released. I imagined Dr. Amony as a dodgeball player, lithely avoiding hurtled lawsuits like so many light red air-filled balls. When they left, I retrieved the charts for my group patients from the nursing station and wrote notes in each, as T. had instructed: "Mr. so-and-so attended morning therapy group."

Group had been almost full that morning, five patients, three of them new to me. Mr. Bonture was still there, as was Mr. Younger, the man with the crumbs. "Would you each like to introduce yourselves?" I asked my group. They agreed that they would not.

"I shouldn't even be here," said a toothless older man in

pajamas. "My old lady threw a plate of food at me yesterday, and I'm the one who gets locked up. Women are the source of all problems."

"Not true, it's men," responded a young woman wearing a backpack. Her face had more acne than I'd ever seen on one person. "I just went out with a guy who was so cheap. All he bought me was a cup of coffee and pack of cigarettes, and he told me I owed him. Do I owe him?" she wondered aloud.

"No," said the middle-aged man. "He only wants sex."

"I don't do that," said the girl.

"Relationships don't work, because God isn't in a relationship. Can I leave now?" asked a young guy with eyes too wide who had been reluctant to come in the first place.

"I'd rather you stay. You obviously have things to contribute," I said encouragingly.

"I shouldn't even be here," he responded, walking out. Mr. Younger followed him. He did not have crumbs on his face today, but his button-down shirt was wide open, yet another indication, I thought, that he was not ready to go out into the world.

As I sat in Dr. T.'s office working on my notes, Rhoda came in looking for her. T. was still with the woman who should've just called animal control, so Rhoda sat down to wait, eager to chat. I felt amused and vaguely flattered. Staff did not generally go out of their way to speak to interns at any length. We were so temporary and uncomfortable.

She seemed poised to tell me about herself. "How long have you worked here?" I asked. She smelled like cigarettes, and I guessed that it had been a very long time.

"Sixteen years," she said proudly.

"Do you enjoy it?" I asked.

"I hate it, but the benefits are great. I get free dental," she said.

We both fell silent. She thought some more. "But it's an interesting place. World famous. People in South America know about it. When they need treatment, they fly into JFK and take a cab straight here. They give fake Brooklyn addresses. It's a city hospital. We can't turn anybody away. Doctors all over the country know about G Building. A lot of them rotated through here. They all hated it, too," she declared, her face brightening.

T. returned and was cross with her. "You're distracting my intern from her notes," she said.

"I'm done," I said.

T. picked up a chart and read it, then another. "These have no substance," she declared. "You cannot simply write that a patient attended and said x, y, or z. Talk about what they are managing to do interpersonally. Note changes in functioning from the last group. In Mr. Younger's chart you write that he left the group after five minutes, but I don't know how long he stayed the day before—maybe five minutes is an improvement. Also, I saw him in the hallway. His face was clean. Say that today he was adequately groomed. We're always keeping discharge in mind, and our notes show whether patients are progressing toward it.

"And what I'm saying doesn't just apply to the charts. Bring these things up with your patients. Once they've been to group a couple times, you can ask them to reflect on how they're getting better. Tell Mr. Younger that you're happy to see his face is clean, and highlight that as a sign of improvement. Then you can ask other patients if they know what 'getting better' looks like for them. Most of them have been here before, and they should start to observe this stuff in themselves."

By Friday, I was like a summer marathoner in her final mile. I also felt back to square one. There were five patients in EOB, and three of them declined my offer of group. A slow-looking woman named Sylvia was alert but unresponsive, and feeling uninterested, I quickly moved on. The two men in the EOB room refused to get out of bed. I let them both know that their refusal would impact their discharge, but they were unmoved. There was an old lady in the private room reserved for the elderly and others unable to protect themselves. When I asked her to come to the dayroom for group, she moved so slowly I decided we'd be better off having the two-person group in her room. After consulting Kelvin to make sure I wasn't breaking rules, I invited my other new charge, Marcus—yet another strapping, young, apparently lucid man—to come into Miss Old Lady's room. He obliged. She was incensed.

"It's not proper to enter a *female's* room," she said to him. He looked at me.

"It's okay if you have a chaperone," I said.

She looked down her nose at me, over her glasses. "In *black* culture, this is not appropriate." I felt chastised for my whiteness, but I couldn't get around it, as glaring and obvious as my inexperience. Maybe they were one and the same. Marcus, whose skin was a good two shades darker than Miss Old Lady's, got up a little irritated with her and stood in the doorway. Group was brisk.

I wrote notes in the two charts and sat to wait for T. Then I got restless and wandered into the hallway, where there was more clamor than usual. The door to Dr. Brink's office was open, and she was seated at her desk. I walked over and inserted myself in her doorjamb. An announcement came over the PA system: "Code Orange on G-51, Code Orange on G-51." Code Orange was an encrypted cry for help, and when it was called, the hospital police and the techs were supposed to drop what they were doing to dash to the offending unit, but the announcements came often, and the staff tended to saunter more than scurry.

"It feels a little crazier here today," I said to Dr. Brink.

She nodded her head with a grave look on her face. "It's the weather," she said. "Changes in barometric pressure make people irritable and explosive. They've done studies."

Dr. T. arrived as if on cue and saw me talking to her nemesis. "What are you doing standing around chatting?" she barked. "There's work to be done." She moved in a huff to her office, and I followed her. My supervisor's quick temper had little effect on me, and this was a delightful surprise, a reminder of one accomplishment of my own therapy: I did not imagine her bad mood any fault of mine. In the parlance of my field, I was not using her crankiness neurotically.

"You should be calling the families after group. Tell them they have to come in and see us. We need to get a sense of each patient's baseline functioning in order to know how much better we can expect them to get here." She took a chart from the stack on her desk. It belonged to Sylvia, the female patient who had not responded to my lukewarm group request that morning. "She lives in an adult home. She went to the hospital for swollen feet, didn't get her Ativan, and became extremely anxious. Call her caseworker and ask her to come in."

Feeling self-conscious under Dr. T.'s gaze, I picked up the phone and called the group home. Sylvia's caseworker would come right over. Sylvia sat with us in T.'s office to wait, still alert but unresponsive. Dull. But when the worker appeared at T.'s door, Sylvia beamed and jumped to her feet. The tall, pretty caseworker smiled broadly as Sylvia threw her arms around her. Suddenly my own lack of interest in this woman who was, if only briefly, my patient made me feel regretful and uncompassionate. The ER was filled with nothing if not raw emotion, which seemed to either hit me too hard or escape me entirely. "Sylvia's always quiet and keeps to herself," the caseworker confirmed for us. T. took the woman's word that Sylvia was ready for discharge. Her caseworker would wait for the paperwork to be complete and then take her home. After they left, T. told me: "Being sent upstairs can be traumatic, so we want to avoid it if the patient really doesn't need it. The psychiatrist wanted to admit Sylvia yesterday afternoon, but Nurse Higgins knows her and thought she'd be okay after she got her meds. This is how it goes here when everything's working as it should. A lot of the patients are familiar to us, and that can be so helpful. We begin to be effective as a community." She paused to let me absorb this information. "Who would you like to see next?"

I told her about Marcus, who had said during group that the police had brought him to CPEP the night before for play fighting on the corner with a friend. "Do you think the police in New York City have time to give a lick about innocent fighting on a corner?" she asked me. I said that seemed unlikely. "It doesn't make any sense," she said with a sigh, forever troubled by my naïveté. "Go get him."

Marcus was still in his pajamas, clutching a pair of jeans. His outfit hadn't seemed strange in the disarray of the early morning, but it was now way past breakfast, and the pajamas felt embarrassing.

"I was just messing around on the corner," he told T. once he was seated in her office.

"That doesn't make any sense," she said, shaking her head.

"There was some alcohol involved," he said.

"How much?" she asked.

"A couple beers," he said.

"That still doesn't make any sense. But we'll come back to it. I want you to tell us about your life."

"My life?"

"Yes. What do you do every day? Do you have a job? Go to school? Do you have friends? A girlfriend? How's your relationship with your family?"

Marcus was twenty-six and did not have a job, had not worked in five years. He had finished high school but did not do any college. His best friend was killed—"in 1997, no wait, it must've been 2007"—by a rapper he seemed to expect us to have heard of. He did not have a girlfriend. He lived with his sister in the same housing project as his mother and stepfather, whom he used to have a good relationship with, "but now there's this thing they won't help me with."

T. asked: "This thing they won't help you with?"

Marcus looked at her. I thought I saw a flash of suspicion, but then his face went blank. "It's nothing. They're very helpful."

"I'm confused. You just said they aren't."

"What do you mean?"

T. tried a different tack. "Why aren't you working, Marcus?"

"I want to work. I haven't been able to find anything. I don't want a minimum-wage job."

"Everyone has to start somewhere," she said. "You're drinking too much to hold down a job."

"No," he said.

She raised her eyebrow. "I want you to go out there for a while and think about all this. Think about why you're here. Be as honest with yourself as you can. And then you're going to come back in, and we're going to have another conversation."

When Marcus went back to the hallway, T. said: "He's not just your run-of-the-mill alcoholic. He's paranoid. He's vacuous. We're not going to learn enough from him about what's going on. Call the family." She flipped open the chart, found a number for Marcus's mom, and set it down in front of me. Graduate school had not required such phone calls, and not for the first time Dr. T.'s full attention left me acutely aware of my unpreparedness. Had my classmates done things like this on their externships? Had the other interns? I imagined they had each performed a hundred brilliant inquiries with families of psychiatric patients and that I would simply never catch up.

I called Marcus's home number and reached his stepfather, who sighed heavily after I identified myself. "Please don't let him out. He'll wind up right back there. He was at Interfaith a couple weeks ago. They said he doesn't have any mental problems, but they're wrong. He's a wild man when he drinks, and he's not right when he's sober either. His mother's terrified he's going to get himself killed, and I don't blame her. We live in a housing project, and he threatens the other young men when he's drunk. He's gotten himself shot at twice. He tried to punch out a cop. His brother just went to jail. My wife can't take losing another boy." The stepfather told me he would bring Marcus's mother in when she returned from her errands later that afternoon, around three o'clock, he guessed. I hung up the phone and conveyed the information to T.

"So what do you think?" she asked me.

I thought in my head. Then I thought out loud. "There are some things in talking to Marcus that don't make a lot of sense."

"Right," she said.

"How he wound up here, for one. Why he's not working, for another. He's only got a high school degree and no work history to speak of but seems to think he's above working for minimum wage. He seems suspicious of his family, and then he got suspicious of you for asking about them. He got the year his friend was killed confused by an entire decade, and then, I guess his friend could have been killed by a famous rapper, but it doesn't seem entirely likely. And his stepfather, the things he said about Marcus picking fights, oh, and that he hasn't managed to get dressed yet this morning."

"What does that all add up to?"

I was stumped. I spoke slowly. "Any one of those things on its own could be explained away."

She shook her head. "No. No, no. We don't explain things away here. We do exactly the opposite. When something doesn't make sense to you, that's the thing to zero in on. Use a telescopic lens. If it doesn't make sense, it doesn't make sense for a reason. Something is not right. I imagine the police picked up on it, or they wouldn't have brought him here. And this is not his first hospitalization besides. Anyway, we're going to keep him for a couple days. I think there's some kind of psychotic process, maybe schizophrenia. We'll have to observe and talk to his mother. Can you come back later this afternoon?"

When I arrived at three, T. was waiting. "Mrs. Stevens's husband dropped her off. She and Marcus have been talking for a few minutes. Go get them and bring them in," she directed.

Like all of the mothers and other visitors I'd seen that week, Mrs. Stevens looked overwrought. She was all but wringing her hands as she sat in the waiting area, looking tiny next to her sturdy son. I led them around the bend and back to Dr. T.'s office. I felt like T.'s lackey and I liked it, absolving me, as I felt it did, of any real responsibility. Marcus and Mrs. Stevens took the chairs. I returned to my perch on the desk.

Dr. T. looked at them. Mrs. Stevens extracted an envelope from her purse and handed it to my supervisor. "I wrote this," she said, nodding. T. took a typed letter out of the envelope and put it down on the desk so she and I could read it together. It was addressed to a judge, and it implored him to commit Marcus to rehab. The letter was heartfelt. In it Mrs. Stevens struggled with formality, as if enough multisyllabic words could convince this magistrate of justice and thereby save her child. But Marcus had committed no crime, and so there could be no sentence, and all the best grammar would not fix whatever was going awry in this young man's mind.

"One problem, though," said T., "is that he's not functioning even when he's sober."

His mother began to cry. "That's true," she said.

"Alexandra!" exclaimed Marcus, addressing his mother by her first name, his frustration palpable. "I haven't done anything! I haven't even done anything!"

"Exactly! You don't do anything!" she exclaimed. "You sit around your sister's house. You drink. You get the people around you angry. This is not a life!" His mother took a tissue from T.'s desk and wiped her eyes.

"How do you process what your mother is saying to you?" Dr. T. asked him.

"She hates me. She's always so critical of me," he said, sounding enraged, looking at the floor.

"Did he tell you about his friend who was shot this year? Did he tell you about his brother? Did he tell you about all the times he's almost gotten himself killed?"

"It's nothing! You're making a big deal out of nothing! Everyone makes such a big deal about nothing!"

Mrs. Stevens was crying harder now: "How can you call your life nothing?"

Marcus jumped out of his chair, towering over her. "Alexandra!" he implored. T. was up, too, in a flash, her hand gently on his chest.

"Marcus, enough." She was firm. "Out in the hall! You need to cool down. Out." She opened her door and Marcus followed her orders, tense as he crossed the threshold. T. watched him walk away and begin to collect himself before she closed the door.

"How long has he been like this?" T. asked Mrs. Stevens.

"He started drinking about five years ago. But like my husband told you, he's not right even when he's sober. He's suspicious of us. Won't let anybody help him. Then his friend was shot to death on the street, and his brother—he worshipped his older brother, and now he's gone, too. Prison. Twenty-five years." She looked up at us, not crying anymore, just relating facts and challenging us to accept them as she'd had to.

"He's had a lot of trauma," T. told her. "Trauma impacts different people differently depending on how they're wired. How it's affected your son is that he's become withdrawn, he's retreated into himself, he's severed his connection to reality somewhat, though that might have happened even without these difficult circumstances, we can't really know. I'm going to admit him upstairs as soon as there's a bed. He'll stay for a few days or maybe longer, until they can get him stable on an antipsychotic medication. He'll be encouraged to come for outpatient treatment after he gets out, and you can support him in that. But it has to fail before it can work. For people with the kinds of problems I suspect Marcus has, it generally takes between three and five years between diagnosis and actually sticking with treatment."

"He doesn't have between three and five years," said Mrs. Stevens, still matter-of-fact: angry young man plus bad neighborhood plus psychosis equals short life expectancy. It was heart wrenching, and I was barely holding back tears—not for the patient, who had not taken in the gravity of his situation, but for the mother, who had. T. sighed.

"We can't know, yet, how this will play out," she said.

Mrs. Stevens went out the front door, and it was time for me to go too. But I left and I didn't. All weekend long I dreamed about the ER. Fragments, not narratives, and when I tried, I could not even convey anything coherent about the dreams. Still I knew, when I awoke unrested, that I had been in CPEP as I slept, among the unquiet minds.

CHAPTER FIVE

WHILE MY MORNINGS WERE SPENT IN THE PSYCH ER, MY afternoons were filled with other pursuits, or in pursuit of having other pursuits. If I lived in a world where people who weren't in therapy were suspect (beyond just my classmates, most of my New York City friends saw therapists, it was just what one did, like going to the gym), in East Flatbush the opposite was true, and getting anyone who wasn't locked up to come see a psychologist required at the very least a handful of phone calls, and then another handful after that. This aversion to treatment had a lot to do with shame. Somehow coming to see a therapist was the worst thing. Perhaps as a corrective, and also because this was the fashionable attitude, Kings County's Behavioral Health department had taken the stance that difficulties in living were "illnesses" that developed in the body, without having much to do with context: if you were "sick," it wasn't your "fault." That life was more complicated than that nobody bothered to get into.

Upon discharge from the G Building, former inpatients were often referred for treatment to the outpatient clinic, the N Building. Once registered there, they were assigned to Phase One, psychoeducation. In rooms with desks and chalkboards, they were then educated in groups about their so-called medical conditions. Divorced as these supposed illnesses became from any possibility of non-medicinal assistance, was it any wonder that afterward patients with profound difficulties relating to others saw little point in beginning Phase Two, group psychotherapy? This was clearly the first obstacle for the women in my depression group, only one of whom was showing up regularly. When the other women did come, they called what we were doing "class." I was also seeing a family headed by a mother who'd been similarly undereducated about her teen daughter's problems, and they were failing to appear more often than not. It was certainly my responsibility to engage my patients in treatment, and I was trying, but the cards were stacked against me at the outset by the very institution that was supposed to share my goals.

The frustrations of the N Building quickly revealed themselves to be stymieing. The chart room there was a Stone Age quagmire staffed by a cranky matron. It was her job to retrieve patients' charts from the high shelves—indeed, getting them oneself was prohibited—but she acted as if she were doing an enormous favor when she took a request and then was as likely to fulfill it as not. The psychiatry residents who worked in the clinic, prescribing medication to the outpatients who managed to show up, were as unenthusiastic as the chart room lady about working with the psychology interns. We'd been paired up with these residents early in the year, the idea being that we would collaborate on the same case—the interns doing the talk therapy, the residents doing the medicating. "Collaboration" was the operative word, as Scott presented this as a peer relationship, a chance to learn from each other. We were all, as it were, trainees. The residents—who had their own director of training, and God only knows what he'd said to them—didn't see it that way.

"She needs some cognitive-behavioral therapy," my resident instructed me sternly as I sat down in his office for the first time. He was talking about Carmen Thompson, my paltry single individual outpatient. Neither of us had met her yet, though we'd both read her chart.

"She needs 37.5 milligrams of ProzacXanaxWellbutrin!" I wanted to exclaim, but instead I just asked him what made him say that.

"She has cognitive distortions," he said, getting up to dismiss me. This resident was very busy, and giving vague orders was all he had time for. It was our first meeting, and then, too, it was our last.

The other interns had longer encounters with their residents, but with similar outcomes. In the quiet of our own office, Leora related a conversation that actually went like this:

Resident: You need to set an agenda for your patient in each session.
Leora: That's not how I work.
Resident: Well, you should.
Leora: Listen, why don't we stick to our own areas of expertise?
Resident: And what are those?
Leora: I know more about therapy. You know more about medication.
Resident: No. I know as much as you about therapy. I know more about medication.

What else was there to be said?

All of these cognitive distortions aside, once I finally met Carmen Thompson, I found her effervescent and flirtatious (character style: hysterical). She liked a rapt audience for her stories. But early traumas suffered at the hands of a withdrawn mother and an abusive father had left her terrified of intimacy, which might have developed with any of the four intern therapists before me had she ever managed to show up consistently. She'd been coming to the N Building for five years, since before the advent of this phase model, which had been put in place only recently to solve the problem of understaffing—it took fewer therapists to treat people in groups. Carmen had been grandfathered into individual therapy, which I gleaned was only still an offering in N to give us interns the opportunity to conduct it. It was as if these patients were to be our playthings in this anachronistic endeavor we called psychological treatment. Carmen was as casual about coming to her therapy as the N Building was about providing it.

Just as my supervisor the neuropsychologist Caitlin Downs had warned, Carmen had been hard to pin down from the beginning. When she didn't show up for our first scheduled appointment, I went directly to Caitlin's office to suggest delaying our first official supervision, which was supposed to take place the following morning. "I figure since I haven't seen her yet, we won't have anything to talk about," I said. I had never opted out of a supervision before: there was always something to talk about with a well-schooled therapist. But after our initial frustrating discussion, I was already uninterested in Caitlin's thought process, and the idea of spending forty-five minutes with her at a stretch, even with a session to present, was taxing. Without one I didn't think I could bear it. Caitlin granted my request but looked dubious and put off.

"Should I not have done that?" I asked the other interns later.

"Well, you haven't seen the patient yet, so it doesn't seem so bad," said Alisa, who was always putting a kind spin on things. But I would keep doing it, every time Carmen canceled thereafter.

When Carmen and I finally met for our first session, I described it to Caitlin unenthusiastically the next day, not out of lack of engagement with Carmen, who like all patients was plenty interesting, but out of the hopelessness inherent in the supervisory situation. I'd concluded that Caitlin had nothing to offer me. It wasn't her fault. She was a neuropsychologist. I might have gotten over this and tried simply to enjoy her company, but I was cranky in the wake of what felt like multiple disappointments, and also Caitlin, taking umbrage at my obvious indifference, was refusing to make herself enjoyable. Soon Carmen had called once more to cancel.

"I told you so," said Caitlin the next time I saw her. "If you had brought cancellations up like I told you to the first time we met, this wouldn't have happened."

But of course it would have. Patients don't stop acting out just because they're instructed to. If it were that easy, no one would need therapy. I explained this to Caitlin tolerantly, but she didn't seem to appreciate the lesson, or the others I delivered later and with less forbearance after her pronouncements of points I deemed similarly misinformed, until we were barely talking about Carmen at all. Forced into a corner by the unfortunate combination of our respective personalities, Caitlin made it clear that she was to be the supervisor here—there was no room for my two cents. I took the hint but chewed it up and spit it out at her, and then I did it again. By the end of a handful of meetings her frustration with me was as clear as my impotent rage. We would go on like that for some time.

- - - - - - - - - -

Marcus Stevens—whose mother had lost first one son to jail and now maybe this one to the G Building—was not quick to leave the psych ER. On his fourth morning there he joined me for group, along with a Mr. Williams and a Mr. Roberts. The former sat and stared eerily. The latter was talkative: "Everyone here is watching me. Why are they watching me?"

"What are you worried about?" I asked.

"They all hate me," he said. "Please tell them not to hate me." He was dressed from head to toe in camouflage fabrics: cap, oversized T-shirt, nylon gym shorts. For some reason, maybe because of the lull in professional attention that came along with the skeleton-staffed weekend, non-EOB patients kept wandering in asking if they could be a part of the group. Dr. T. had told me the answer to that question was no, and I tried to enforce it, but sometimes people just sat down to listen, and truly I didn't mind, because it made me feel sought after.

Marcus said to Mr. Roberts, "Don't worry so much what other people think of you."

"Why so quiet, Mr. Williams?" I asked, trying to bring our third member into the discussion.

He tensed up. "I'm trying to control my anger," he said quietly, concentrating hard. I nodded in response, chilled by his gaze. He went back to staring straight ahead.

After group Mr. Roberts told me he felt much better than earlier in the morning. The contact had apparently done him some good. I told that to Dr. T., adding that it was nice to hear but that I still didn't feel as if I was doing much in group.

"Well, you go back there every morning and try. That's something," she said. Her praise was always tepid, but no less than I felt I deserved. "Just remember, you *can* be therapeutic," she encouraged. I asked her about the notably intense look on Mr. Williams's face.

"It's called the psychotic stare," she said. Then, "When someone tells you he's struggling to control his anger, ask him, 'Do you think it might be hard to control it here today?' and 'What can we do to help you?' You also have to tell the staff. He may need to be assigned an assault level so that we know to keep a close eye on him.

"With Mr. Roberts, probe his paranoia. Why does everyone hate him? Are there reasons people would want to watch him? Is his family connected to this? The CIA? Explain that the staff is looking at him because it is their job to take care of him and make sure he's doing okay.

"So, now. We have a new admission. I want you to interview him. Remember the telescopic lens. You want to know what brought him here—the presenting problem, and also the history of the presenting problem." She nodded and went to get this new person. When she returned, she was accompanied by a tall, hefty man in his mid-forties wearing a flannel shirt and pajama shorts. "This is Miss Lockman," said T. by way of introduction. I winced at the title: unlike my first name alone, it served as an explicit reminder that I was not yet a doctor. I wondered if the patient felt shortchanged. His first chance to tell his story, and all they offer him is a "miss."

"Henry," said the man, nodding at me.

He did not look crazy. If colloquially speaking there were more or less two categories of patients here—suicidal/homicidal or totally nuts—it was my guess that he fell into the former. T. sat down in the third chair. I was in charge.

"Can you tell me what brings you here today, Henry?" I asked, disconcerted as always under Dr. T.'s scrutiny. When I was only recounting to my supervisors what I'd said and done in sessions, at least I could leave out the parts I'd deemed most egregious. Here, in situ, my most ridiculous moments—as certain to manifest as the morning dew—were so public.

"I was thinking about killing myself. I brought myself here instead."

"Did you have a plan?" I asked.

"I've been staying with my brother. He's got a lot of pills in his house." He waved his hand, et cetera, et cetera.

I nodded, thinking. As a journalist, I'd asked questions for a living, and that suited me—the coaxing of a linear narrative, the culling of the insubstantial details. If only Dr. T. were not sitting there, this would come so much more naturally. I tried to think of the right next question. "What's been going on in your life that got you to this point?"

"I lost my job. I'm frustrated. I'm tired. My family is at a distance."

"What were you doing for work?"

"I was in waste management for four years, picking up Dumpsters."

"Were you laid off?" I asked.

He looked at me, weary. "I got fired. I wasn't going in all the time. I was stressed-out. I have too much to do. For the past couple of months I was missing work two or three days at a time. I was so tired."

"Why do you think you're so tired?"

"I don't know."

"Do you have trouble falling asleep or staying asleep?"

"No."

"Can you say a little more about your family? You mentioned they're at a distance?"

"Yeah, they say they've had enough of me. That's not how family should be. My brother is better. He took me in three years ago. I've been living with him, but I've decided to leave. His girlfriend is pregnant, so it's time to find a place of my own."

"You're going to miss living with them?" I asked, trying to glean some sort of cataclysmic loss or injury from his story. He seemed sort of down, but I wasn't hearing or feeling anything that added up to suicide.

"They've been good to me. But I can see it's time to go," he said.

"They kicked you out," announced T. Her statement felt jarring against my gently spoken inquiries.

"If you want to look at it that way," he said, his back up.

"How many years have you been using?" she asked, and I understood that T.—having had enough of me missing the obvious—was taking over.

"Fifteen or twenty years. What of it?" he asked.

"Alcohol?"

"Heroin, crack, alcohol. Check, check, check." He was sarcastic now.

"How much?"

"Two hundred dollars a week on heroin. A six-pack a day."

"When was the last time you used?" T. wanted to know.

"Yesterday," he said.

"How many times have you tried a program?"

"I just left my fourth," he said.

"Did you finish?"

"I took a break. Went to jail for a while. Disorderly. Pos-

session. I got out, and I went back to the program. Left again."
He was blasé now, not proud of his habits, but maybe of his
defiance.

"Do you think that's why your family is done with you?"

"Probably." He was nodding now.

"And that's why you were too tired to make it into work?"

"I suppose so."

"So what's your biggest concern right now?"

"Housing," he said. "I need a place to live."

"Well, I guess you've got that here." She smiled a thin,
tight smile.

"I don't know what you're talking about. I'm depressed. I
want to kill myself," he said with no real feeling.

"You've alienated everyone in your life," said T. loudly.
"Your family, your employer. The brother who stood by you
longer than anyone else doesn't even want much to do with
you anymore, and yet you don't seem to care."

He just looked at her. I vaguely remembered learning
that this was the hard tack one was supposed to take with an
addict, but I'd never worked with any. Conventional wisdom
held that therapy did little good with active substance abusers.
Drugs and alcohol interfere with the brain changes associated
with learning and so progress in psychotherapy. I never quite
understood, though, how an active drug user was supposed to
get sober without the help of a therapist from the get-go. Was
the yelling intended to facilitate that? When he left T.'s office,
I asked her.

"With an obvious drug addict, it's all about straight con-
frontation. It's the only way to begin to cut through his denial.
He's full of shit, and you tell him as much. Suicidal, give me a
break. He wants a place to stay. This is better than a shelter."

"So do we let him stay?" I asked.

"He's already been admitted to EOB. He'll spend one night at least. Tomorrow you'll have another chance with him. You can practice being confrontational."

The next morning I led three patients into the group room only to find an obese man sitting on a chair against the back wall masturbating. From the doorway I told him that he had to leave, but he was not all ears. I asked a passing nurse for help, and she tried what I'd done, telling him from a distance that it was time to go. He ignored her, too. I wondered what Dr. T. would do. If it was part of my job to tell grown men to wipe crumbs from their faces, was it also my responsibility to let them know that public displays of autoeroticism were frowned upon? If one needed to be told, was it not a moot point? The nurse summoned the security guard nearest to us, a woman who suggested getting the two male guards from the waiting area to deal with our problem patient, who by the by was not on my list. The officers were summoned and led the man out of the room. My charges stood waiting, nonplussed. In what I imagined were gestures of equal parts solidarity and self-preservation, the patients rarely batted an eye at their peers' most outlandish behaviors. I turned off the television—how much easier that part had gotten—and began group.

Henry was there that morning, along with two other men. I asked each to explain what he was doing in the psychiatric emergency room. Henry said that he'd wanted to kill himself, and also, with a snicker, "It's going to be cold out soon." The second man said that he wanted to kill his family, and the third that he wanted to kill his boss.

"So you three have something in common," I said, growing ever more comfortable with feeling slightly ridiculous. "You all came here in order to stop yourselves from doing something damaging and irreparable."

After group I invited Henry into T.'s office. She wasn't in yet, and so I could carry out her order—"practice being confrontational"—with only Henry to bear witness to my folly.

We sat down. "You mentioned in group that it's going to get cold soon. I took that to mean you plan to use the hospital as your winter home?"

"No," he said. "I just want to get better." He grinned. He'd inferred I was a trainee, that I'd been naive about his game yesterday, and that he'd been used to teach me a lesson. Now he was going to have some fun at my expense.

"Are you feeling ready to leave?"

"No," he said again. "I'm comfortable here."

"Well, you're not crazy, and you can't stay," I said firmly.

"But if I leave, I might kill myself."

"You might overdose on heroin," I said. "But the treatment we do here is not what you need."

"I need another program?" he asked. He'd dropped out of so many already. I could hardly feign enthusiasm about another.

"I imagine you need to stop using drugs, to go to work every day, to regain your family's trust."

"Maybe," he said. "But right now I'm too busy being in denial." With this he was smirking, making fun of me and all that I was aspiring toward. I felt ashamed and thought about how that feeling might be related to his own, and then yelling at him just felt beside the point, the continuation of a thousand humiliations he'd experienced over decades.

"You act like this is all a joke, but it doesn't really seem very funny," was as confrontational as I could be. Henry gave me a look to let me know I was boring him. I opened the door for him to leave. Rhoda came by. "T. said to tell you she had to go to a meeting. She said there's an interview for you to do. A Mr. Cook. Young guy. He got here around three a.m. Cops brought him in for making prank 911 calls. One of the residents just evaluated him and admitted him to EOB."

I found Mr. Cook sitting soberly in the waiting room. He was in his mid-twenties, African American, in expensive pressed jeans, a short-sleeved orange Polo shirt, and flip-flops. He was better groomed than any of the patients I'd seen and also some of the staff. Hope fluttered familiar: maybe there was nothing wrong with this one. Mr. Cook was polite and composed when I brought him in to Dr. T.'s office and shut the door behind us. "Why don't you start off by telling me how you got here?"

"The police," he said. "They got angry at me for calling them, so they brought me here. I suppose to punish me." He looked at the floor, shaking his head.

"Why were you calling them?" I asked.

"I've been having a dispute with my across-the-hall neighbor. We used to be friends. She's old and she can't work anymore, so she's always broke, and I used to take her out to dinner sometimes. We leave our doors open when we're both home so my dog can wander back and forth. I lent her twenty-five dollars a few weeks ago, and ever since she's been avoiding me. I wanted my money, so I decided to wait for her outside her door. She got home at three a.m., and I was there, so she called the police."

"She called the police just because you were standing there?"

"Well, I'd been bothering her about the money for the last week or so. I think she kidnapped the cat I was cat-sitting to get back at me. Anyway, I wouldn't let her get into her apartment. I was insisting she give me the twenty-five dollars."

"What did the police do?"

"They came, we were both still standing there. I told them what she'd done. They told me to go home, to take it to civil court, and they left. But after they left, she threatened to stab me, so I called 911. The same cops came back, more irritated this time. They were going to arrest me, but instead they brought me here."

I felt sympathy for the plight of these beleaguered cops, but did they really need to bring this nice fellow to a psychiatric emergency room just to teach him a lesson?

"Have you ever been in the hospital before?" I asked.

"No," he replied.

"Have you ever been involved with the police?"

"No, never."

"Have you ever seen a psychologist or a psychiatrist?"

"My wife and I went to couples therapy a few times, before our divorce."

Couples therapy? Only functional people went to couples therapy. I was sure of it. This guy was fine. The police were only human. Sometimes they retaliated, like with the lady with the squirrel. No harm, no foul.

I did what I'd learned to call a mental status exam. Mr. Cook knew who and where he was. He did not hear things that other people couldn't hear. He could identify the president, and the one before him. He did not think the television was talking directly to him. He was sleeping regularly and eating heartily. He could count backward from a hundred by sevens. I racked my brain for what to do next and remembered Dr. T.'s lesson about leaning on people, going hard at their judgment to see if it pushed them over the edge.

"You can't just wait outside a woman's door at three in the morning and then refuse to leave. You're going to get yourself in real trouble," I chastised him. "You can't act like that in the world."

"I see that," he said. I felt relieved. His response was so normal. He would take in my words, and he would stop behaving so ridiculously. I had talked some sense into him. Phew.

I told him he could leave the office. That we would meet again later. I wrote a chart note and prepared to tell Dr. T. that I thought it was true this time, that someone had messed up, that this person really did not belong here.

"It's not that easy to wind up in the G-ER," she said with exasperation when she returned and I gave her my take on Mr. Cook. "Did anything in his story *not* make sense to you?"

"A lot of little things were slightly off," I admitted.

"Like what?" she asked.

"Well, this is New York. No one lends money to a neighbor, or leaves their apartment door open to let their dog wander in and out. I mean, maybe if he was romantically interested in her, but he said she's old, and she must be a bit crazy, too, if she really threatened to stab him. And then there was the thing about the cat kidnapping. I mean, it's possible . . ." I trailed off.

"But not likely," finished T.

I thought aloud: "I'm finding that I work really hard to organize what patients tell me. I push the stuff that's bizarre to the back of my mind and focus on what does make sense."

"Why do you think you're doing that?"

"If I let the stories *not* make sense, I feel off-kilter. It's disorienting."

"So you have a tiny taste of how psychosis might feel," said T. "That's good. You're very empathic, exactly what we all need to be. Pay attention to how hard you're working with any particular patient to organize their experience. It can be a signal to you of how *dis*organized their thought process is. Bring Mr. Cook back in."

This time I found my patient just to the right of T.'s office, standing on his head. He righted himself and followed me back to the small room. When Dr. T. asked, he told us more about his life. He worked as a telemarketer. He had a college degree from an online university, though he'd spent his first two years of undergrad at Cornell. "You know what they say," he told us, "the easiest Ivy to get into and the hardest to graduate from." He'd gotten divorced because "we fought about money. Couples often fight about money." His mother had died one year prior, and he told us calmly, "I went through the stages of grief."

After he left, Dr. T. asked what I thought once again. I said, "He was behaving bizarrely when I went out to get him, standing on his head in the hall. It's strange that he started at Cornell and finished at some Internet college. And he seems smart, but he works as a telemarketer."

"He doesn't have to have any face-to-face contact with people that way," she said. "His affect was very flat. That's what stands out to me. He answers questions about emotions with abstractions. I think he's trying very hard to sound conventional when it comes to talking about feelings."

"So you think he's schizoid?" I asked, testing the waters with T. by referring not to a psychiatric disorder but to a character style, a descriptor for someone whose fears about closeness keep him isolated, who doesn't experience his emotional world the way other people do, who's interpersonally a bit odd.

"Probably," she replied. "He generally gets by. Nobody on the street would know anything was off."

"So what do we do for him?"

"The police thought something was wrong. Taking that

into consideration, we'll keep him and observe. We'll make sure that his judgment isn't a threat to his safety. He is likely schizoid, but he may also be headed toward the more psychotic end of that spectrum. He could be having a first break. There's no family to call for collateral information, though maybe he'll agree to let us talk to his ex-wife. With a patient like Mr. Cook, you wait a bit and see."

The next day I was off. I took an "education day," as opposed to a vacation day, to meet with my dissertation adviser. We went out to the very end of Long Island, where we courted the social psychologist whose data I was hoping to mine. Over lunch in the food court at SUNY Stony Brook we discussed research measures of adult attachment and their relationship to psycholinguistics, and by the time I returned to the psych ER the next day, Mr. Cook was gone, sent upstairs, and I never saw him again. That was CPEP for you. Blink and you'd miss someone, or maybe a patient would be there four weekdays straight, and you'd feel as if you'd lived out her harrowing course alongside her over many months. On my day away, immersed in the minutiae of academia, I relished the conversations of people unalarmed by the exigencies of the emergency loony bin. Was that the real world? Was this? They were so disparate that going back and forth between the two was viscerally unnerving, like jumping from the hot tub to the cold pool at the Russian baths.

Too soon I was back in my morning group, with a young white drug addict brought in by—"BIB" in chart shorthand—his sister. There was a young, pretty black woman who'd asked her husband to bring her in after watching "upsetting events" on the news; one man who wouldn't say why he was there at all; a tearful young woman with no front teeth to whom I paid less mind than I might've because of her appearance and the fact that she lived in a group home; and an oddly dressed thirtysomething whose "affect was not appropriate to content" when he reported, with a grin, that he was there for beating his caseworker. After group I called the purportedly clobbered caseworker. She laughed and said that no, he wasn't violent, just not med compliant, and I guessed that I must've been the biggest believer of nonsense who'd ever crossed the CPEP threshold with her very own skeleton key.

The next morning, the same patients were still there, and we felt like old friends, or I felt as if we were old friends for all of us. This helped me relax, and probably not coincidentally they were the most interactive group I'd led. Mr. Fincher—the white drug addict who lived in an affluent Brooklyn neighborhood not usually inhabited by Kings County patients—explained, as if it were no biggie, that he'd disappeared on a crack binge for a week and his mother and sister had flown in from Phoenix to find him on the streets and bring him to the hospital. Mrs. Kendrick—who'd been upset by the television—told us through her tears that she was responsible for some gang killings of teenagers she'd seen on the news. In actuality, she had nothing to do with gangs, but it is common, in psychosis, to believe oneself at the center of events literally—if not psychologically—unrelated to you. Shirley, the toothless woman I'd considered so uninteresting the day before, had found herself an ornamental headband and a denim miniskirt, and her mood was brighter and her attitude more confident, and she strutted around the group room as if she were one of the Supremes; she interrupted the others as they talked, and I had no patience with her. The man who wouldn't speak the day before was now talking enough to share that he was waiting for a bed upstairs, and the one who'd claimed to have beaten his caseworker said he was going home later that day.

Group lasted twenty-five minutes—a good ten longer than usual—because of Dr. T.'s insistent voice in the back of my head: you can be therapeutic. I waited for something to inspire me, but for all of the interesting content, nothing did, and group ended with its usual whimper.

When I got back to T.'s office, there was a note from her. "Went to meeting. Fincher's mother and sister will be here at 11:00 to take him home. Talk to him—the hard line—and then to them—limit setting." The day before, I'd been in T.'s office as she spoke to the young man's mom on the phone. The mother had asked, "Is he still mad at me for bringing him in?" and T. had almost lost it. I got Fincher from the hallway and brought him into my room. In a Yankees cap and with two days of stubble, he did not look particularly interested in anything I might have to say.

"So your mom and your sister are coming to pick you up."

"Great," he said.

"You don't sound like you mean that."

"They're the ones who brought me here. I didn't belong in the first place. My roommate never should have called them."

"What do you think would have happened to you?"

"The same thing as always. I wind up back at my apartment, living my life."

"How long do you think you can go on like this?" I asked. This was not his first crack binge, his first disappearance.

"Until I get tired of it. Then I'll go back to school. I'm going to be a psychologist."

"What makes you interested in that?"

"I'm good with people," he said.

"Psychologists have to spend a lot of time working on themselves. Did you know that?"

"I don't need any work," he said.

"You're in a psychiatric emergency room. As a patient," I reminded him.

"I didn't need to be here," he reiterated.

Dr. T. had instructed me exactly what to say. In a stern voice I managed: "You've just lost another semester's tuition. You're twenty-six, and you've barely finished a year of college. You're not going anywhere until you stop using drugs. Certainly not into a doctoral program," I added, sounding harsher than I felt.

He looked at me angrily. "What's the point of this?"

I cringed. I had asked T. the same thing. She reminded me, "Because someday, when he's ready, he'll remember what you said and it may be of use to him."

I told him, "You're not ready to truly look at yourself yet. Someday maybe you will be, and you'll remember what I've said." I was not even convincing myself. I hadn't said anything particularly profound. He was going to be a burnout, and a corpse waiting to happen, until he stopped using crack: like, duh.

"Are we done here?" he asked.

When I went to get Fincher's mother and sister from the waiting area at 11:00, they were upper-middle-class and white and so at once felt immediately—wincingly—familiar to me. As we settled into T.'s office, I relaxed in a way that I had not managed in CPEP in all of my days. My unease there was so multifaceted I hadn't quite connected it to the differences in class and race that were almost constant givens for me in the setting, but now, as I melted into T.'s chair, it was startling in its obviousness.

The room fell silent. Mrs. Fincher looked clueless and out of place. She wore a large diamond ring on her index finger, and her dark hair was blown straight. She had on a brave face, but it didn't feel like the right one. The sister was another story. Her eyes were bloodshot, and she looked as if she hadn't slept, and I thought of my own sibling and how I might feel under similar circumstances. I recited the short speech Dr. T. had prepared for me.

"You need to stop coddling him," I said. "You need to set limits. Trying to be nice and rescuing him is not going to help him get clean."

"That's what everyone has told us," Mrs. Fincher said.

"Right," I said.

"I don't understand," intoned his sister with intensity. "Am I just supposed to sit back quietly and let my brother kill himself?" She was enraged. Mrs. Fincher put a hand on her daughter's back. I wished I had an answer that could make it even a little better, and I half believed there was one.

Afterward, as I told T. about the brief meeting, I surprised myself by bursting into tears. Though my eyes regularly teared in response to sad stories, the bursting was another matter. It came on like a sneeze, but with less warning. It was notable, and it was the second time in my life it had happened. The first had also been in supervision, during graduate school, and my supervisor back then had hypothesized the tears really belonged to the patient I was discussing, who'd appeared to feel nothing as she detailed a childhood filled with unthinkable neglect. Was this that? The idea suggested a certain emotional contagion addressed by theory—a patient's split-off feelings are communicated nonverbally to the therapist, who can unconsciously process them and give them back in less potent form, like a mother bird chewing food for her chick. But I also had my very own preexisting despondent feelings about difficulties I was powerless to affect. What of this bursting was about the Finchers, and what of it was about me? That was always the unknowable thing.

T. handed me a tissue and waited. I wasn't sure what part of my thinking to share. I saw there was little time, in a psychiatric emergency room, to contemplate the esoteric questions of graduate school outpatient treatments. "Things move so fast here you never get a chance to process how you feel. I think it's been building up. I'm sorry for the tears."

"Never apologize for having an emotion," T. said. "Just make sure you give it some thought."

"My sister lied to the police and told them I pulled a knife on her."

"My boyfriend called the police for no reason and told them to bring me here."

"My wife is the one who needs help. I called 911 and asked them to bring me here to set an example for her."

"I had a couple beers and thought I wanted to kill myself, but now that I have no more drink in me, I'm feeling good, and I have no reason to be here."

Such were the collection of stories that began my mornings. By week three I had conquered the patient roundup and the television, finally to find myself dealing with actual psychological problems—rampant externalization and denial.

T. instructed: "When the whole group is blaming someone else for why they're here, say, 'I find this hard to believe. All these doctors here are so stupid as to admit you for no reason? They want to make you all suffer while the real bad guys are out there going about their lives?'"

"I've been asking them to think about what's going on inside of them, rather than what's going on outside," I told her.

"No," she said. "Too sophisticated. Say to them: 'None of you have any problems?'"

"They'll say they don't," I said glumly. That particular day I had run what felt like a pronouncedly stubborn and self-defeating group.

"Then say, 'Okay, well, I guess we'll just have to agree to disagree.'"

But I was also getting sharper. When a patient I had been indulgent with during group said to me, "You understand me so much better than Dr. T.," I knew right away that he was a substance abuser and that I had missed this issue and Dr. T. had not. For the rest of that day, each time he saw me in the hall, he told me that I should get a raise. Actually, the opposite was true. The next day, T. and I spoke to him together. T. asked him if he had any thoughts about what they'd talked about the day before. He could not remember the conversation.

"I think it had something to do with your drinking," I told him. He never mentioned my raise again.

Of course each time I felt satisfied with my growing competence, there was something to remind me of how little I knew, if not about my field per se, then certainly about the world. One morning Rhoda presented me with a Mr. Rain, thirty years old and unwashed. "He was brought in for threatening to shoot someone at his new group home," she told me.

We went into T.'s office to talk. He was gentle and truly not smart. He told me that he hated his new residence. I asked if he thought he had any alternatives. "I was in foster care once," he said. "I liked it. Can I go back there?"

After Mr. Rain and I finished, Rhoda came in to ask

whether he had access to a weapon. I didn't know, because despite his presenting problem I hadn't thought to ask and the very idea that he could have obtained a gun sounded preposterous to me, which I didn't hesitate to tell her. She didn't hesitate to look at me as if I were an idiot.

"This is East Flatbush! You can get a gun on any street corner!"

There were other things you could get on Brooklyn street corners that I didn't know much about either, but I learned about from people like Mr. Tacks, who had been quick, in morning group, to let me know that he didn't belong in the psych ER. During group, Mr. Tacks's story concerned calling the police in order *to set an example for* his wife. It changed when I sat with him one-on-one. "I called them *to come take her away*, but then I realized she needed to be home to watch our daughter, so I went instead," he said.

"That doesn't make any sense, Mr. Tacks." I liked that line, it was so knowing and world-weary. I'd stolen it from Dr. T.

"What makes no sense is keeping me here. I've got multiple businesses to run, and being in here just keeps me from making money for my family. I've been away long enough. I just got back from upstate in May. My businesses are suffering." He spoke quickly and a little too loudly and was having more fun than anyone deserved to have in the psychiatric emergency room. Sure, mania had its downside, but it could also be a hoot.

"What did you go upstate for?" (I felt so satisfied, knowing he meant prison.)

"Assault," he said. "It was my fourth incarceration. My second or third there was a corrections officer who disrespected me. Me and my boys went and found him. They beat the guy. I waved around a gun, decided not to shoot. We showed him." He puffed out his considerable chest.

"But you went to jail for . . ."

"Four years," he said. "And I'm taking names of people who piss me off here."

I took a deep breath. A danger to others, possibly. Poor insight and judgment, for sure. "So what you're saying to me—someone who works here—is that if you get angry at any of the staff members, you will track them down and hurt them? Do you think that assault is a good idea? Do you think that telling me of your intentions is a good idea?"

"What are you talking about? I didn't say that."

After we were done, Mrs. Tacks had come to visit, and I brought her in with him to get a clearer sense of why her husband was there in the first place. "The last time he was hospitalized was at Elmhurst ten years ago. They told him to call 911 if he ever needed help. He woke up from a post-beer nap feeling depressed and called EMS. I told him not to do it," she said. "Now he's stuck here for a while, right?" I informed her he'd been admitted for seventy-two-hour observation. She continued, "I called the police on him last week for putting his hands on me. He slapped me, and they took him away, but actually I hit him first. It didn't look too good for him," she said, pointing to her rounded belly. She was notably pregnant. She continued, "He got back from jail seven months ago, and just like that we're having another kid. I have two older kids, but our first daughter together is four. I had her while he was away. He didn't even know about her until he got home."

Mr. Tacks was quiet for a change. "Why did you hit him?" I asked her.

She gave him a dirty look. He said, "She's so jealous. I went out to the store, and she thought I was with another woman."

"How long was he gone?" I asked her.

He answered before she could: "Five minutes."

"Has he been unfaithful to you in the past?" I asked her.

"Yes," she replied.

"We weren't together then!" he said to her, and then turned to me to explain. "When I got out, I slept with one of my hos."

My eyes opened wide, and I didn't bother to try to hide my middle-class surprise. "You're a pimp?" I asked him.

"Not anymore," he said.

I took a deep breath. "What goes on between the two of you that things get so heated that you're hitting each other?"

He brushed me off with his right hand, apparently incensed by the question: "I'm a shooter, not a hitter."

Mrs. Tacks was no more abashed about her own antisocial tendencies. "I held up a bank once with my asthma inhaler. They gave me money, and I never got caught." Again I was stumped. My silence unnerved her: "How else was I supposed to feed my kids?"

T. laughed when I recounted the meeting. "Your typical narcissistic-borderline couple," she said. Narcissists, who have a fragile sense of self that they bolster with grandiosity, often pair with borderlines, who are likely to provide them with the idealization they crave. "Who else did you have in group this morning?"

I listed the names, forgetting the toothless woman and then remembering. "Oh, and Shirley."

"She's going home today. We should see her first. Why do you think you almost left her out?"

"She lives in a group home. She doesn't have any front

BROOKLYN ZOO

teeth. I think I see her and assume she's a hopeless case, so I end up being more focused on the other patients. Also, she was interrupting the others a lot. I felt really annoyed; it's so hard to get a conversation going in there, and she was making it harder."

"Don't be so quick to dismiss her as un-helpable. Teach her something," she said. "Ask the other group members to talk about what it's like for them when Shirley interrupts. She may not get it now, but it will stay with her. We know Shirley here. We see her and other people like her over and over. The staff starts to get frustrated. I'm no exception. Just last week I saw Sequoia Diaz and rolled my eyes, thinking, 'She's back again!' She used to come in every month. And I saw her, and it was obvious I was exasperated, and she said to me, 'But, Dr. T., it's been almost eight months!' And it had been. She said, 'I've been trying, but it's hard!' So I told the staff to congratulate her on going almost eight months between ER visits."

I found Shirley in her miniskirt and her headband and asked her to come to T.'s office. She was so friendly toward me, and I felt guilty for my indifference toward her over the past three mornings. As Dr. T. and I spoke to her, Dr. Amony came in to wish her well, which I had never seen him do with any of the other patients. In his suit and his accent he was as dignified as a head of state, and I thought that Shirley was a valued customer, and I saw that it made her feel good. "Be calm at your residence," he told her, serene but stern.

I walked Shirley toward the front to meet her caseworker, who would take her home. Shirley was so excited she tried to hug me with a toothless smile. "No touching!" I said reflexively, feeling like an insensitive jerk but also not wanting her fleshy bosom pressed against mine. I stuck out my hand to shake hers instead, which of course involved touching and

143

might have been confusing. She asked for my card. I hoped her request meant that she hadn't noticed my coldness, though it would have been better, for her own good in the world, were she able to pick up on others' signals, no matter how rejecting. At any rate, I didn't have a card. I apologized.

When there were only two EOB patients and one refused to get out of bed, I did not have a group. I asked a Miss Williams, who was standing in the hallway peering over her shoulder, to come into T.'s office alone. She was my size but with a psychotic stare intense enough that it left me cold inside. I kept the door to the office open as we sat down because one of the few things I'd learned in grad school about working with psychotic patients was that their delicate sense of safety was predicated on being able to flee. I also made sure her chair was closest to the door. She was fragile looking and rather beautiful, if not so well-groomed, like a television actress made up as a crazy person for a role. She had light brown skin and haunted amber eyes.

I began with simple questions to see how disoriented she might be. She knew the date, the day of the week, the name of the hospital, and even that we were in the G Building.

"How old are you?"

"Twenty-three," she responded. Her chart said thirty-nine, and she looked it.

"What year were you born?"

"Nineteen thirty-one." Which would have put her in her mid-seventies.

"How far did you go in school?"

"I finished seventh grade and then got a scholarship to the college Parsons School of Design."

"Sometimes when people are having problems like the kind you're having, they hear voices that other people can't hear. Is that happening with you?"

She glanced at me furtively and did not respond. I tried again.

"A lot of people who come here tell us that they feel down. They have trouble eating and sleeping. Is any of that bothering you?"

She didn't answer in words but drew away from me a little, staring straight ahead and beginning to rock back and forth.

"Are you feeling afraid of me?" I asked, again rather scared myself.

She nodded, and I told her the door was open and that she could leave if she needed to. She got up and tiptoed out and then from outside the office asked me for some water. I told her I'd walk with her to the nursing station, where we could get a cup. We moved slowly down the hall next to each other, and she asked quietly if I could also get her some crack. "I do crack every day," she said.

"That's very sad, to do crack every day," I said, because it was the first thing that came to my mind.

"What are you talking about? I don't do crack," she replied.

After I'd gotten her some water and we parted, the frightened feeling stayed in my body for quite a while.

Sometimes when I did not feel fear, I felt loathing. Laverne: I even hated her name. She was all baby fat and at twenty-six had just given birth to her fourth crack-addicted infant, whom the Administration for Children's Services had quickly relieved her of. The intensity of my feelings toward her tipped me off that her developmental level was not psychotic but borderline, meaning that while she'd achieved the tasks of the first year of life (basic trust, and faith in the fact of her existence), she'd had some trouble with those of the second (separation and individuation, or knowing that one is a separate person from one's mother and beginning to establish a distinct identity). Borderlines rely on the same primitive defenses as psychotics, but their reality testing is better. They see the world in more conventional ways. While psychotic patients tend to stimulate benignly parental and empathetic feelings in their caregivers, borderlines are famous for enraging those around them. Hence my loathing, though it was of course not solely her doing, as nothing can be aroused in you that doesn't already reside there.

"Are you going to help me get my check?" Laverne asked T. She was dressed in a hospital gown and no bra, and her postpartum breasts were pouring out the sides. Often there were too many exposed body parts in the psych ER.

"That's not my job here," T. responded, managing to maintain a sympathetic tone. "I'm here to help us figure out what's going on with you."

"What's going on is that I need my check."

"Why did the ambulance bring you here, Laverne?"

"I called them," she said.

"How come?" asked T.

"I didn't have carfare," she replied.

"You told the admitting psychiatrist that you felt depressed," T. began.

"That's irrelevant," Laverne declared.

"I don't think so," said T.

"Why would I care what you think? Last time I was here they helped me get my check. That's what I want."

"There are social workers here who will help you with the life issues you need help with, but our job right now is to try to get to know you a little, to learn about your life."

"That's irrelevant," Laverne said again.

T. persisted, but Laverne was not interested in doing any reflecting. My supervisor finally gave up and sent her out in the hallway.

"You're so patient," I said when Laverne was gone. "I could barely stand to be in the same room with her." ("Neither could her mother," my professor's voice repeated in my ear.)

T. said: "Developmentally, she's a baby. You wouldn't get angry with a baby. With a patient like this you need to find some leverage. She wants child services to let her see her newborn. We'll let her know that they're going to read her records and that she needs to cooperate with us if they're going to give her what she wants."

The next morning Laverne was on me the moment I raised my illicit key to Dr. T.'s lock. "Are you the one that's doing my discharge?" she asked. She was dressed in jeans and a tight pink sweatshirt under a fitted denim blazer, and for a moment I didn't recognize her. I hated her less when she was clothed, all of her parts contained. "Laverne? I barely recognized you. You look great!" I said to her, remembering T.'s directive to help patients begin to recognize their own improvements. I told her that I didn't think she was being discharged but that we could talk more in group. For the second day in a row there were only two EOB patients, but they both agreed to attend, and the three of us—Laverne, Mr. Roy, and I—made ourselves cozy in the TV room. Mr. Roy was around Laverne's age. I asked them to talk about why they were there. Laverne said that she'd been depressed but was better now, and Mr. Roy said he was schizoaffective, which Laverne didn't know about.

He explained: "It means I get depressed and also hear voices. Mostly God's voice, but I've learned to live with it."

After group I got their charts to make entries. I read over Mr. Roy's, my attention caught by a nursing note from earlier that morning. It seemed Mr. Roy had complained that he was awoken at 6:00 a.m. by Miss Williams—the woman with the chilling stare. She was bent down over his pelvis, her mouth clutching him. When T. arrived, I told her what I'd read. She said she'd just come from talking to Nurse Higgins about the whole thing. "Probably true. Whatever happened, she went and hid in the restroom afterward, in the tall garbage pail. A patient went in there to pee and saw her intense little eyes peering over the top of it. He ran from the bathroom screaming." In the aftermath, Miss Williams had been admitted upstairs. T. was on her way to try to smooth things over with Mr. Roy's mother, who was threatening to sue the hospital. Between the patients and their families, someone was always threatening to sue the hospital, the understandable fallback position of the irate and disenfranchised, who then didn't always bother once the anger had receded. I brought Laverne in to talk.

"I need to know a bit about your life and your background," I told her. She told me that she'd moved in with her most recent baby daddy the day they'd met one year earlier, but that there'd been "infidelity."

"He cheated on you?"

"No. I needed money for drugs."

"So you prostituted yourself?"

"No. I had male friends I knew would give me money."

"For sex?"

"Yes," she said.

She told me she'd been raised by both of her parents until her mother died of AIDS when she was fourteen, at which point she was on her own.

"What about your father?" I asked.

"I never knew my father!" she yelled. Everything that came out of her mouth had an angry lilt. She went on to talk about wanting to get off drugs, about getting her baby back. I asked how she planned to do this.

"I'll wear an S on my chest like Superwoman," she told me, full of bluster.

T. came back as we were talking. "When am I going to get my discharge?" Laverne wanted to know from her.

"You have to show me that you can think. That you can plan," said T.

Laverne picked at her fingernails. T. told her to leave. "Come back when you've thought about what I said," she said.

Some time later T.'s door was open, and Laverne wandered in eating a sausage and cheese biscuit that someone must have brought her. She addressed us only by burping loudly. "Can you say excuse me?" asked T.

"Excuse you," Laverne replied sassily.

After she'd wandered back out, T. said: "Her sarcasm is a sign of intelligence. It's obnoxious, obviously, but it's also encouraging."

The next morning Laverne refused to come to group, but there were three new patients in the EOB, plus Mr. Roy, who remained. One of the new patients, an older man, was wearing a lot of layers, shirt on top of shirt on top of vest on top of robe. I called his residence—a nursing home—after group. These calls had become a regular part of my morning. What was the patient's history? What was his baseline functioning? I spoke with the social worker there, who asked, "Is he wearing lots of tops? If he is, he's still out of his mind and not ready to come back."

None of that morning's patients were ready to leave. Mr.

Roy was still psychotic, or at least I guessed as much from his report during group. "The hospital police woke me in the middle of the night and got in my face and called me a bitch," he said.

"Why did they do that?" I asked, imagining that they had done nothing of the sort.

"I don't know," he said, looking confused.

"Do you think you were dreaming or hallucinating?" I asked.

"Maybe," he agreed, nodding. I took his ability to consider my suggestion as a sign that he was emerging from his psychosis and noted the entire exchange in the chart, as Dr. T. had been encouraging me to do.

The two remaining patients were the most interesting to me: Mr. Rumbert, because he was selectively mute, which I hadn't yet encountered, and Mr. Jean, who was lucid and sad, which meant we could have a good conversation. I brought Mr. Jean into T.'s office first. He was nineteen and in the ER after making a suicidal gesture.

"What did you do?" I asked him. The admission note had been hard to read, which wasn't unusual.

"Pills," he said. He was in a football jersey, tall with light skin, cornrows, and acne. "Adderall, Tylenol, Zyprexa." I knew by now that the latter was for serious psychiatric problems—bipolar disorder, schizophrenia. His age made me guess he'd been recently diagnosed.

"How come?" I asked.

"My mother. I live with her. She's crazy. She calls me a piece of shit. She said she wished I was dead, so I ran into the bathroom and started shoving pills in my face." He began to cry. I handed him the box of tissues on T.'s desk, and he took one, blowing his nose loudly.

"She really gets to you."

He nodded, continuing to cry. I sat quietly, feeling bad for the guy, saddled as he was with such a horrible mother. T. walked in on the middle of our tears and sympathy.

"What was going on that your mother got so angry with you?" she wanted to know.

"I don't know," he said.

"You don't know?"

"She's just like that," he said. T. suggested he spend some time in the hallway reflecting on how he had contributed to his troubles with his mother. The hallway: our version of a think tank. When he was gone, T. had me call the errant mom.

"He goes wild in the house when he gets upset, and he's set off really easily," she told me calmly. "He throws things at me. Breaks things. I had to retire last year because of my health. I can't take his behavior anymore. It's too much."

When we hung up, I repeated the information to Dr. T., who nodded. She'd heard the same story a hundred times, if not a hundred thousand.

"I just felt so bad for him," I told her. "My feelings distracted me. I didn't challenge him, because it didn't occur to me that his mother could be anything but crazy." (An unfortunate artifact—there were so many—of my treatment-resistant desire to condemn my own mother, to exonerate myself.)

She looked at me hard. "You react strongly to the patients." She didn't seem to mean this as a compliment.

"I know," I said. "Is that unusual?" The overpowering resonance of others' sadness in my soul was as automatic to my being as the heavy way I walked, and I usually forgot it was particular to me, or to others with similar psychological structures. But besides that, the ER was such a raw environment, I'd assumed it roused strong feelings in everyone,

T. included. For weeks I'd been chalking up her exaggerated sharpness to the emotional stresses of her job, to the constant burden of digesting the unprocessed madness that surrounded her on her own personal western front. I couldn't believe that in some gentler reality, my teacher would remain so resolutely shrill.

"People respond differently. But you should always look at it," T. said. "Have you tried therapy?"

- - - - - - - - - -

The ER was crowded, the line for meds twenty people deep, and I waited for my morning patients with impatience. "Fifty-four total on the census today. It's too much to handle," Rhoda said to me when she saw me waiting. "Bellevue's psych ER never takes more than twenty, even though they have five times the physical space as us and twice the staff." I asked her about the discrepancy. "Because it's in Manhattan and because they get white patients," she said.

Rhoda wandered off, and a rare and manic white guy in his forties came and stood beside me, talking as fast as one of those fast talkers on a TV commercial, but he was not limited by thirty seconds of airtime, and it was truly impressive, his ability to go on and on and on at that speed and not stop. With fifty-four patients, no one was getting enough attention. After the distribution of caplets and capsules and liquids, I ushered my six into the dayroom. Mr. Jean was still there and still stewing about his mother. Mr. Rumbert remained selectively mute. A pretty Indian girl who was new to me had a now familiar psychotic stare and was also choosing not to speak. Despite the fellatio incident, Mr. Roy lingered. When group ended, I returned to T.'s office to record our proceedings faithfully in the charts. T. came in and shut the door behind her. She did not sit down. She was short of breath.

"What mistake do you think you made when you wrote in Mr. Roy's chart the other day?" she asked me, her backside pressed against the door as if to prevent me from leaving. Her tone made me nervous, and I couldn't for the life of me remember what I'd written. I didn't have it in front of me, because Mr. Roy's chart had been missing from the nursing station when I'd collected the others.

"Refresh my memory?" I asked reluctantly.

"Hospital police, getting in his face, calling him a bitch."

"Oh." I began to sense where this was going, and I felt a little dizzy. I explained, "But obviously that didn't happen. I wrote it down because he agreed it was a hallucination. I thought that showed he was making progress, like you've been teaching me." My voice tapered off.

T. moved away from the door and sat down in the chair next to her desk. "Dr. Amony just read what you wrote. He was reviewing the chart because it's on its way to administration because Mr. Roy's mother is threatening to sue over the blow job. Do you see what the problem is?"

I did not want to, but I did. She continued.

"A lawyer reading that chart does not understand psychosis. He does not understand delusions and hallucinations and paranoia. He only understands that his client made a serious allegation against the hospital police and that the staff dismissed that allegation without even bothering to ask anyone who'd been on duty the night before what might have happened."

"Oh," I said. I was an imbecile. There was no way around it. My contributions to CPEP were meager, especially compared with the price the hospital might ultimately pay for inviting me to complete my training there.

"Would you like to know how you should have handled the situation?" T. asked.

I did.

"If you were ever again to note something like that at all—and there are many reasons you might decide it was better not to—but if you did, you have to investigate. To follow up and see whether there was anything to what Mr. Roy was claiming. I agree with you that it's unlikely that this happened. The hospital police are not sadistic, and it's hard to believe that they are arbitrarily waking patients in the middle of the night to call them names. But you cannot record such a thing in a chart, which is first and foremost a legal document, without following up. And by the way, you should have followed up on this whether you chose to record it or not. Maybe something happened with another patient. Who knows? Whatever the reality, it needs to be clear to us."

I nodded again. "I'm so embarrassed," I told her.

She nodded. Her face relaxed, and she softened her tone. "Yes, but you are here to learn, and you certainly won't forget this. Anyway, for the rest of your time here you still need to write notes, because you need the practice, but you will no longer be writing them in the charts. Neither will any of the other interns when they rotate through here, Dr. Amony's orders." I wondered if it would be possible to pass what remained of my time in CPEP without seeing the man. I took some comfort in the fact that he might not connect my face with my crime. T. continued. "Everyone's on edge around here these days. You know about the big lawsuit?" I nodded.

"Mostly just what I read in the *Post*," I told her.

"The hospital's own legal service is suing. Basically, one

of their lawyers got paranoid and started busting in on patient interviews to ask questions and make demands. Dr. Amony kicked him out. The lawyers he worked with got angry and suspicious in return and started actively soliciting ER patients for complaints about their treatment. The most sociopathic patients. The Department of Justice has been called in to investigate. There'll probably be some helpful changes around here as a result, but the staff are on eggshells, trying to make sure everything is in order." T. paused and brushed her hands of the whole matter. "Who should we see first?"

- - - - - - - - -

"What's the date?"

It was not an extraordinary question, but its asker made it so: the young and handsome and well-groomed Mr. Rumbert, from Barbados, had not uttered a syllable since he'd arrived in CPEP three days earlier, and now here he was with a complete sentence. We'd spent several groups together, and I hoped that his attendance had contributed at least a little to the end of his mutism or at least to the fact that he had chosen me to speak with. "Mr. Rumbert! You're talking today! You must be feeling so much better." My enthusiasm was intended to impress upon him, as Dr. T. had taught, what it meant for him to improve. I told him the date was October 26.

"I thought it was some—" He stopped abruptly and stared at me with concern. We were standing in the hallway outside T.'s office.

"What is it?" I asked.

"It's your eyes," he said. "I'm not sure if maybe they could zap me." I assured him they could not and asked him to come into the office to chat. As we were getting seated, T. arrived. I began the interview.

"You're so much better today. Do you have a sense of why?"

T. cut me off with her hand. She looked at me. "Too complicated," she said. She turned to Mr. Rumbert. "Did you get breakfast?" she asked. "You haven't been eating."

"It's hard to eat because I can't leave. It's like I'm in prison," he said.

I started, "This isn't a—," only to be cut off by T.

"Does he know where he is?" T. asked me quietly. I asked him.

"It may be a prison. I'm not sure," he said. His accent was refined. Slightly English sounding.

"You're in a hospital, sweetie," said T. He pondered that information. "Why don't you go out and have a seat and think about that?" she suggested, but Mr. Rumbert stayed where he was. T. began to do paperwork, and he sat and watched, trying to figure out if she warranted his trust or his suspicion. T. left with some papers in hand, and Mr. Rumbert and I remained in the office. He turned to me.

"You remind me of a character on a show on the Sci-Fi channel," he told me. "The guy on the show is trapped in this village, and people try to convince him of things. You look like one of those people."

"You're worried that I want to convince you of something that's not true," I interpreted. "Me and Dr. T."

He laughed. I looked at him, puzzled.

"It's her name," he said. "It's funny."

I woke a woman named Ophelia for morning group, and she was not pleased. "You woke me from my sunder," she kept repeating in an angry voice. She followed me into the dayroom anyway. A man named Juan was dancing in the hallways, and I corralled him, too. There was a third patient, a woman, she looked a little slow. And Mr. Rumbert again. I asked them to speak about why they were in CPEP.

"I came for a bed, but I was double-crossed," said Ophelia.

"My fiancée called 911 after Shabbos dinner," Juan said, which sounded funny because he was clearly Mexican.

"Why did she call?" I inquired.

"You'd have to ask her," he replied.

The woman who looked slow said she'd done crack for the first time and was full of regret. She began to cry.

Rhoda walked in to get Ophelia. She needed her help with some paperwork.

"You can come back when you're finished," I told the patient as she left. She turned and gave me the finger. Juan told those of us who remained that he wanted to read to us from a book called *Recreating Your Self*. As we listened, Ophelia returned, and she was worked up. She marched up right close to me.

"You double-crossed me," she yelled. Her body looked tense, poised for a fight. For the first time in the ER, my fear of being physically threatened was being realized. I made my way toward the door, encouraging Ophelia to come with me, not wanting to leave her alone with the other patients. She was taller than I was, and wiry. I imagined her rage would give her fists great force. I had never learned how to protect myself from a punch, and cowering seemed like my best defense. I remembered what T. had told me weeks earlier about being soothing.

"It's okay. Come with me. We'll find you some juice, something to eat," I said. She followed me as I walked backward into the hallway, which for once was deserted, the guard having abandoned her post. Ophelia remained too close, still menacing, insisting on my alleged crime, taunting me. I continued walking slowly, my body facing toward her as I backed away sideways. "Hello, hello," I said loudly, turning my head toward the adjacent halls, trying to get the staff's attention without alarming anyone, but someone was always yelling, if not screaming, in the ER, and no one was likely to heed my cautious cries. Calling for help seemed overly dramatic, and I thought it might set Ophelia off besides. Shit.

But Rhoda came out of her office and saw us. She rushed over, inserting her solid body between Ophelia's and mine. She managed to calm her down while also explaining to me that Ophelia had slammed out of her office two minutes before. "I'll take care of you," Rhoda said firmly to Ophelia, shepherding her off to another hallway. I went back to the group room, concerned that the patients might have gotten spooked. Juan and the other woman were now seated side by side. She was choosing passages from his book, and he was reading these aloud. Mr. Rumbert sat across the room, silent but calm. I entered and closed the door and sat to listen and get myself back together. Ophelia was back soon, standing outside the windows of the group room looking in. I saw the guard was back at her post, and I opened the door. "Would you like to rejoin us?" I asked Ophelia, because wasn't that my job?

"Don't talk to me," she said. "You look like a canker sore."

Afterward, I did not have much left in me, but still I brought Juan into T.'s office for an interview. His chart said he had a long history of bipolar disorder. He told me he was an attorney and a converted Jew and there was no reason for him to be in a psychiatric emergency room.

"Have you been hearing voices?" I asked.

"Yes," pause, "Guided by Voices," pause. "Get it? The band?" Guffaw.

"Are you worried that someone is watching you?"

"Yes," pause, "the Police," pause. "Every breath I take, every step I make."

He kept insisting there was no reason for him to be there, and when T. came in, she'd quickly had enough and told him we were done. He got up and walked out, turning off the light as he made his exit.

"That's so symbolic," T. said. "Lights out." I told her about what happened with Ophelia because I thought the staff might want to assign her an assault level. T. asked if I was okay. I was still shaken, but I said yes. Then it was time to go, and as I left, I saw Juan the converted Jew lying on his stomach on one of the reclining chairs. I waved, and he thrust his hands back to catch his ankles in a resplendent yoga bow pose.

All the way to work the next morning I debated whether to bring Ophelia to group. I hadn't thought to ask T. about that. With a higher-functioning patient—someone who was not psychotic—I thought it would have been important to bring her in, to demonstrate implicitly that her aggressive impulses were not as destructive as she likely feared. I was not sure that the same thinking applied to a psychotic patient, especially a paranoid one, since paranoia reflects a projection of aggression—that is, Ophelia experienced the hostility not as her own but as directed toward her by those around her (in this case, me). I decided I would invite her if she was up but that I would not wake her from her "sunder" if she was still asleep. It turned out not to matter, because when I got the census she was no longer on it—moved to the list of people waiting for a bed upstairs. I was relieved. I found Juan and Mr. Rumbert—who was continuing to speak—and a new woman who was attractive and looked with-it. But then she told me she did "sortation" for a living, which made me suspect she had a thought disorder because I knew, thanks to my month in the psych ER, that use of neologisms was often a symptom of schizophrenia or mania. T. called in sick, and Dr. Brink was my official supervisor for the day.

I spoke to the sortater, who had a long history of psychiatric hospitalizations, for some time and then went to report to Dr. Brink. She seemed distracted, and I felt as if I was bothering her; EOB patients were not her problem, after all, and I didn't imagine her relationship with T. made her inclined to fill in with her caseload. The hospital police were called to the ER while I sat in Brink's office, but I paid that little mind. When I got up to go back across the hall, she put her hand out to stop me. "Didn't you hear that page? You never leave after hearing the hospital police called. You need to pay attention." It had been a month, and there were many things I had learned there, but others that I had not. I sat to wait while the police broke up a fight in the hallway.

The next day was a Friday, and my last in the psychiatric emergency room; on Monday, I would report to inpatient unit G-51. I gathered the EOB patients for my final group with ease. A moment of interpersonal conflict between two group members got me engaged. The drug addict told another patient he didn't like being asked about his methadone in the hallway in front of everyone the previous day. The offender replied he'd noticed the drug addict had not eaten breakfast and was testing a theory that methadone users in general didn't like to eat. I tried to facilitate further discussion, which would have been the meat of an outpatient group, but neither man was as interested as I was.

After group Rhoda told me there was an EOB patient pending. A psychiatrist I recognized by face but not by name told me I should see him to try to make something of his story. Darren looked like a handful of the others I'd seen that month: early twenties and handsome and robust, nicely dressed in jeans and a sweater. His presence in the G-ER didn't bode well, but I was still maintaining my manic hope that somehow nothing was seriously wrong this time. T. came in as I was beginning my interview with Darren and quietly sat down to observe. I felt my usual self-consciousness and also a determination to do better this time, to prove to us both that my four weeks of immersion in her EOB had taught me something. Darren made eye contact and answered my questions in the right amount of detail, without hesitation or mistrust. To make matters murkier, his reason for admission puzzled me, and I didn't know where to go with it. "A week of really bad headaches," he said. If there was one thing I'd learned, it was that you didn't get brought to a psychiatric emergency room for a headache.

"Did the headaches start because you'd been drinking too much or using drugs?" I asked.

"No, I'm not into any of that," he said.

"Did your headache come from voices you were hearing that no one else could hear?"

He shook his head.

"Was it because someone was stealing your thoughts or trying to put ideas into your head?"

He gave me a wry smile. Still no.

"Did the headache make you agitated? Did you get very angry at anyone, maybe yell at them on the street or shove them?"

Negative. We sat there together, equally perplexed.

"Where was the pain?" I asked, grasping at straws. If he told me it was in his face, maybe I could diagnose him with a sinus infection. He said that it was in his entire head. I turned to T., defeated. "Do you have any questions?" I half mumbled.

She took over with her usual omniscience. It was not grandiosity, she just really was all knowing. I tried to calculate the difference between my four weeks and her twenty years. Even allowing for fifteen vacation days annually, it was considerable. "Your thoughts were all jumbled up last week, and it really made your head hurt," she said to Darren. He nodded, and it was as if a light had turned on in his brain.

"They were mad bundled!" he said.

"And that happened in school, too, right? It got hard to pay attention, hard not to get confused?" Darren had told us that he'd flunked out of college four months earlier.

He nodded, starting to look upset. T. had his chart open in front of her and was looking at the doctor's orders. "Has the medicine we've been giving you helped with the headache?" she asked.

"Yes," he replied. "It's gone now."

"You're lucky," she told him. "Years ago we didn't have these pills, and people who got headaches and confusion like yours had much more trouble going about their lives."

After Darren had left us for the hallway, T. said, "Most likely schizophreniform, though it could be a psychotic depression." She explained that schizophreniform disorder was diagnosed in patients with less than six months of symptoms of schizophrenia; only some of them would go on to exhibit the full-blown disorder. "His prognosis is good. He relates pretty normally, and his affect isn't flat. If he stays on the medication, he can probably go back to school, next semester even. He should see a therapist, too, of course, to monitor how he's doing over time, to help him understand his preoccupations better. He's far from a hopeless case."

"How about me?" I asked, aware that my minutes there were dwindling, wanting to remind T. that today it was me who was timing out.

"Not hopeless," she said. "Frankly, I was surprised by how little you knew when you got here. But you've been doing a good job trying to take everything in. It's a lot of information, and it's a difficult environment. I wasn't sure you'd come back after what happened the other day with Ophelia."

This floored me. It never crossed my mind not to return. What kind of wimp did she take me for? "No. I mean, I was shaken, but this is my internship. I signed up for this," I reminded her. She pulled out the same evaluation sheet that Dr. Young had filled out the month before. T. had not given me high marks, but at least they were scores that actually reflected her own ideas about my work. As she reviewed them with me, I thought again about what Dr. Wolfe had said the month before, and how after so long in the carpeted classrooms of my graduate school it was actually quite hard to pull off, this task of becoming a better psychologist. But also I felt on my way.

CHAPTER SIX

ON THE FIRST MORNING OF OUR INPATIENT ROTATION, Bruce and Tamar and I met in the intern office to go downstairs as a group. The other four adult-track interns had just spent sixteen weeks on inpatient together, and their snowballing collection of inside jokes about medical students we'd never met and patients we'd never seen had highlighted for the rest of us the isolation of our solo rotations—forensics and CPEP for me, neuropsych and consultation liaison for Bruce and Tamar, respectively. I hoped we'd develop our own rollicking camaraderie, but despite our affectionate predispositions toward one another the chemistry felt off. Bruce and I had become friends, almost, but he was private and hard to get to know. Of all the interns, he'd also developed the most immediate and astringent dislike for our shared environs, and his crankiness rubbed up against my own and blistered there. Tamar had two kids at home, and when we all convened in our office, its floor now caked with dirt after a rainy October, she was the last to arrive and the first to go. She was kind and good-humored, but being around her tended to make me feel repellently frivolous, like a Valley Girl or someone too concerned with celebrity magazines. I couldn't quite figure out why, though like any good graduate student in clinical psychology I'd tried.

The three of us put down our coats and our bags on six, and then Bruce let us into the dim, concrete stairwell with his skeleton key, unlocking and locking the heavy doors that let us down one flight. We went to the right and through one more locked door to meet Dr. Meyer, our new supervisor, in his small and barren office just outside the unit. Tamar and I took the two seats on either side of Meyer while Bruce stood, chivalrously. Our supervising psychologist was diminutive with a genial smile and a close beard. He was in his forties and didn't seem enthusiastic about the experience we were about to embark upon. "We'll spend most of our time initially talking about paperwork," he told us wearily before going over the admission notes, treatment plans, and discharge summaries we'd be expected to write for our patients. He said we needed to be especially focused on these right now because the Justice Department would be reading them. The paperwork also seemed to be what he expected would most distinguish us on the unit from the other professions. "Before you write a note," he said, "ask yourself: Could a nurse write it? Could a social worker write it? If they could write it, you are not doing your job. We need to carve out a place for ourselves here." (But why, I wanted to groan rhetorically, was it not already carved for us?)

When Meyer finished, he told us it was time to go onto the unit. "Morning meeting," he said. "For the whole staff. Every day, about 10:00." The three of us closed our notebooks and followed him through one more locked door and onto G-51.

On the other side of a bolted door we found six or seven morning-crusted patients lounging dispiritedly around the dayroom, a large, stale-smelling space with the now familiar cold white concrete floors and rusty-paned windows that did not open. In one half of the room were wood-framed sofas of cracking pink vinyl and an old color television console locked in a plastic case. In the other half were six or seven rectangular dining tables with black plastic chairs. Some of the patients stared at the TV, its volume loud enough to be noxious as it reverberated off the cream-colored cinder-block walls. A commercial for a calling card blared the last digits of its toll-free number, "Four, four, four, four." People wandered into and out of the room or sat at tables staring into space or still finishing breakfast. An aisle down the middle of the room led through an open door and into two separate hallways, at the hub of which was a nursing station. The staff bathroom was in the station, and Meyer promised us keys. One hallway housed the women's rooms—each as institutional and aged as the dayroom, but much smaller and with wooden platform beds built into their floors. All you could say for the vinyl mattresses was that they were probably easy to clean. The men's hall was almost identical, with its eight rooms and one dormitory-style bathroom and shower, though it also contained the chart room, where the staff met and where new admissions were interviewed. A few patients were scattered outside its door waiting just like in the ER for the promise of a better day.

Dr. Meyer wore his skeleton key fastened to his pants, as did all the interns by now thanks to my former classmate Leora, who had congenially tracked down and purchased seven identical key clips with elastics that extended easily from waist to shoulder height, where the keyholes in G were set. Meyer used his key now to let our group into the chart room, quickly pushing the door closed with his slight mass and bolting it. Inside and outside might have been separated by a moat. Like every other room in the building, it was dingy, sepia toned. A large, weathered table took up most of the space, and getting past the detritus that surrounded it—stray papers, old computer desks, filing cabinets—took some maneuvering. As we sat down around the table, Dr. Meyer introduced us to the two staff people working quietly there, their backs to the door—Miss Smith, a beautiful older black woman dressed all in red whose fleshy hips were too big for her frame, and Oswald, who was Haitian and in large glasses and also getting on in age. Both were social workers and longtime veterans of the inpatient unit, Meyer told us. They were friendly and welcomed us. We sat down across from them on the far side of the room.

After not very long at all, Dr. Begum, one of the two psychiatrists who ran the unit, entered. A lanky Bangladeshi immigrant, he was middle-aged with dark, thinning hair and a sardonic half smile. Shaking his head, he looked around the small room. "Where is everybody?" he asked with frustration that seemed playful, slamming down his stack of folders, after Meyer had introduced us. Oswald and Miss Smith barely looked up from their work, and my group certainly couldn't answer. Who was "everybody"? Dr. Begum stomped out of the chart room, returning in little time with five other staff members—nurses and nursing aides, I guessed, and maybe a tech. Dr. Begum took a seat at the head of the table without locking the heavy door behind him, and a patient quickly appeared there. "Oh boy," said Miss Smith under her breath with a sigh.

"Marvin Mavin, you cannot be in here now!" asserted Dr. Begum, his heavily accented English giving his enunciation a staccato clip. Marvin Mavin was as old as Dr. Begum and taut, with eyes open too wide. He swayed into the room, the door heaving shut behind him. "I'm havva. I'm havva navva havva," he said, swinging his arms. He looked ready to launch forward, like a rock in a slingshot. I felt the bodies in the room tense along with my own. The man I'd guessed was a tech stood up. So did Dr. Begum.

"Mr. Mavin!" said the psychiatrist. "I promise you that later we will see you! Right now you need to wait outside." Oswald stood up, too, and as Marvin Mavin lunged at Dr. Begum, he and the tech each grabbed an arm and with some force got Marvin out the door, which one of the nurses locked once they were gone. "He got a shot last night. He's out of control. You need to adjust his medication," she said to Dr. Begum. Oswald and the tech came back into the room, unlocking and then locking the door. We could hear Marvin shouting enraged gibberish in the hallway. He pounded on the door.

"I will take care of it," said Dr. Begum, scribbling a note to himself on his stack of papers. He continued speaking over the clamor. "Where was everybody this morning? Every day we meet! This is not optional. I will not take responsibility for this unit—I will ask for a transfer!—if I cannot get you people into shape!" The staff looked bored. He turned to us, the interns. "I have been at Kings County only as long as you. We were at hospital orientation together—I remember you. I came over from Maimonides. I could not believe how badly this unit was being run, and now I am asking new things from the staff. My requests are not being met with enthusiasm." He paused and looked around the room. "I will leave if things continue as they are!" he repeated, waving a finger in the air. No one reacted. He seemed to be enjoying himself, and I enjoyed him in return. He smiled and shrugged and sat down. He turned to Bruce and Tamar and me again and said: "The morning team meeting is very important. We review all patients' progress. We talk about what is happening on the unit. We assign you therapists to the patients; each will carry about five cases. Then we interview any new admissions."

George had started on inpatient at Columbia the month before. On his unit, "community meetings" preceded the treatment team ones. The patients and staff all convened to address problems the former were having with their stays. It gave the patients a chance to be heard, to work things out by relating to others. George was being taught to lead the meetings, as they were apparently standard operating procedure on locked wards. But Dr. Begum didn't mention these, and I guessed they were not among our offerings.

"Nurse Hector, please begin," Dr. Begum said.

The nurse began reading names from a list that resembled the CPEP census, in the same boldfaced font I'd only ever seen at Kings County. It looked mimeographed. Meyer took copies from the middle of the table and handed them to us. With each name someone on the staff chimed in: how had the patient's night been, was he improving, was he almost ready for discharge. Several patients had only recently arrived, including Mr. Rumbert, my selectively mute friend from the ER. The staff did not know him well yet, so I offered what information I had, despite my ever-needling fear that to offer anything might be to overstep some boundary. Was it a student's job to keep her mouth shut? I wasn't sure. "I worked with him in CPEP. He came in not speaking, but he talked after a few days. He's psychotic—confused and suspicious, frightened but cooperative," I said.

"You will take this patient?" asked Dr. Begum. I was happy to. Mr. Rumbert made three. I'd already been assigned two patients—transferred from Leora—before I'd even arrived for my first day. Each of these women had been living in the decrepitude of the unit for upwards of six months. "Not good therapy cases" was all Leora had to say about them. That was psychology intern shorthand for people who had trouble engaging in what felt to us like meaningful work. I had no experience treating psychotic patients, but I was determined to surmount this: I had just finished reading *I Never Promised You a Rose Garden*—in which a talented psychoanalyst patiently cures a young schizophrenic woman—and had high hopes (Dr. Aronoff might have called them grandiose) for what I would accomplish with patients who weren't "good therapy cases." When the meeting ended, I went out to meet my new charges and to find Mr. Rumbert. I walked into the dayroom looking for any of the three. I knew that one was Vietnamese and the other was an older black woman. Asian people were rare in the G Building, and so were old women. I glimpsed the elderly woman first. She had cropped gray hair and bright eyes. She was wearing an overcoat and sitting on a plastic dining room chair that she'd moved next to the unit's only exit, a shopping bag at her feet. It overflowed like a cornucopia with her things—clothing, toiletries, several striped woolen caps. I approached her. "Are you Gabriel?" I asked, thinking that her name was evidence of her earliest experience with careless parenting. Was she once a girl who should have been, among other things, Gabrielle?

"Yes, I am," she said loudly, raising her eyebrows. "Who are you?"

"I'm Darcy," I said. "I'm your new therapist."

"Well, as you can see, I'm on my way out, leaving. So I

won't be needing a new therapist." She pronounced the last word as if it were hyphenated. "Thera-pissed."

"Where are you going?" I asked her. Of course I was unsure if she was actually leaving. Was she delusional? Optimistic? Was there any difference, on this locked ward, between the two?

"To Kingsboro!" she said. "That's where I'm going. Going and gone-ing. They're coming to get me. I'm out of this dump." I didn't know what Kingsboro was, or if it was anything at all.

"Can we talk a little before you go?"

"No," she said. Her tone did not invite argument, and I didn't want to disrespect her wishes, to get us off on the wrong foot were she really staying. But I didn't want to seem rejecting either.

"Okay, well, I'll make sure to come say hello if you're still here tomorrow."

"Okay," she agreed noncommittally, still watching the door. I walked away, in search of Hong Hanh. There were no Vietnamese women in the dayroom, so I headed for the women's hallway. In the second room on the left, I found a tiny, middle-aged woman in red sweatpants and a hospital gown with shoulder-length black-and-gray hair sitting on the room's only bed.

"Miss Hanh?" I asked. Some patients made me want to use their last names. She looked up from her writing. I continued. "I'm Darcy. I'm your new therapist."

"You tell Dr. Win-kler I no need be here," she said with some urgency. Dr. Winkler was the other psychiatrist on the unit. He had not been at the morning meeting, so I hadn't met him yet. The interns who'd just finished up on the unit had described him as old and doddering.

"I thought we could talk a little, start to get to know each other," I said. She looked at me blankly. Good grief. "Do you speak English, Miss Hanh?" I asked.

"No English," she said. "Little English," she corrected herself and stood up, coming very close to me. "You tell Dr. Win-kler?"

"I'll make sure to talk to him," I said, trying to make my voice reassuring because I didn't know if she could understand my words. She sat back down cross-legged on the bed, and I left. What was one more inauspicious beginning among so many? I went to the men's hall to look for Mr. Rumbert. My dejection peaked when I found him lying on a bed wrapped from head to toe in a white sheet. I recognized him only from the shape of his haircut. "Mr. Rumbert!" I was still happy to see him, even if his half recovery in CPEP had been short-lived. "It's Miss Lockman, from the ER!" I hoped he would respond to my joy at our reunion with at least some interest, but he did not move. Who put the catatonia in catatonic schizophrenia? "I'll be working with you while you're here," I told him. "Maybe tomorrow you'll feel more like talking." I returned to the chart room to note my interactions with my patients in language I hoped would carve out a place for my field. As Dr. Meyer had implicitly predicted, my work that day had not.

The next morning I walked onto the unit to find Gabriel waiting by the door again, in her coat and with her bag. "I'm leaving today," she told me when I greeted her. I thought that she recognized me, but she didn't seem to remember that she'd given me the same (mis)information the day before. Was she psychotic or demented or both, and without psychological testing—which would have been done months ago had anyone deemed it important—how would I ever make that determination? Hong Hanh was in the dayroom, too, in the same red sweatpants and with the same old song: "I no need be here. You tell Dr. Win-kler." I clearly needed to know more about these women than they were able to tell me, so I went to the chart room to wait for the meeting and read whatever was legible among their paperwork.

When I unlocked the door, the chart room was empty except for a slim man in his seventies wearing a three-piece brown suit. He had a white beard and a full head of white hair. He was small and handsome. "Dr. Winkler?" I asked. He looked up, and I thought I could hear his neck creak.

"That's right," he said.

"I'm Darcy," I said. "One of the new psychology interns."

"Ah," he said. "Welcome." He emanated a calm I had not felt on the inpatient ward, and at once I realized that the rest of the staff looked on alert—as if afraid they were being followed—all of the time. Zeke and Jen and Alisa and Leora had dismissed Dr. Winkler because of his age and probably something else that I wasn't picking up on yet, but I preferred older psychiatrists, trained in a time when medicine was still interested in the mind as opposed to just the brain.

"Thank you," I said. "I think I'm working with one of your patients. A Vietnamese woman. She's asked me a couple times to tell you that she doesn't need to be here."

He nodded. "Yes, Miss Hanh." He sighed. "She's a difficult case. I'd like for her not to be here, either. She's been declared mentally incompetent by the courts, and her family won't take her in. It's not uncommon for some immigrant families to cast out members who are mentally ill; they can't earn money, so they're a real strain on a family struggling just to survive. She's had a legal guardian appointed who makes decisions for her, and the guardian says she can't go home, even though she owns an apartment. She's been in and out of hospitals. When she got here six or seven months ago, it was after her super saw her place and called EMS. She'd basically turned her apartment into a hovel, took out all the plumbing. I think she was in a refugee camp in Vietnam at some point, probably traumatized during the war, looked like she was trying to re-create that environment. There are pictures in the chart. You should take a look."

"I will," I said. "So does she just stay here indefinitely?"

"We've got her application for Kingsboro in, but a bed hasn't come up for her yet."

"Yes, Kingsboro. What is that place?"

"State hospital. For long-term care. We're an acute care unit, not for long-term stays. We're supposed to be stabilizing patients, preparing them for reentry into the community. When patients aren't going to be ready for discharge within a couple weeks, we're supposed to send them on, but it doesn't always work that way. There aren't enough places for them to go. So we have people like Miss Hanh who get stuck here. It's tragic really."

"So what's my role as her therapist, given that we can't really even communicate particularly?"

"Read her chart. Touch base with her guardian," said Dr. Winkler. "You could try calling her mother or her brother if she'll let you. They're in the Bronx. Last time we called her mother she hung up on us. Her English wasn't good, but I don't think that was why."

"Are you working with Gabriel Nolten, too?" I asked. In addition to having a therapist, each patient on the unit was assigned to a psychiatrist for medication management. Dr.

Winkler and Dr. Begum split the floor, twenty-plus patients in each man's caseload. He nodded.

"She's another one waiting for Kingsboro."

"By the door each morning," I said.

"Yes. The waiting isn't completely nuts. She was supposed to leave last week. After five months on the waiting list, they finally had a bed for her. But she'd turned sixty-two in the time between when we put the application in and when she got accepted. That's the age cap for the adult beds. At sixty-two you need a senior bed. Someone there caught her birth date, and she went straight to the bottom of a different list. No telling when she'll leave now. Her hopes were up. She's not ready to accept it yet."

"What's going on with her?" I asked.

"Long history of schizophrenia, we think," he said. "Lots of psychiatric patients are poor historians. When there's no family to talk to, we're left to do a bit of guesswork. She was brought in by the police after they found her wandering in traffic. She was able to tell us that she'd been in psychiatric hospitals off and on for a long time, and you'll talk to her, you'll see her symptoms."

"She didn't seem to remember that she told me yesterday she was leaving. Could she have dementia?"

"That could be going on, too," he agreed. Others were settling around the table now. Tamar and Bruce had come in and sat down to the right of me. I thanked Dr. Winkler for all the information, and in a flurry of good mornings Dr. Begum called the meeting to order. There was a new patient sent up fresh from CPEP, and after we reviewed the census, one of the nurses went out to fetch him. Dr. Begum turned to the interns. "I will do the interview. I want to know why he's here and also about his history: substance abuse, previous hospitalizations, family, et cetera. I will do a mental status exam, find out about health problems. Many things. Today I will do the interview, but usually I want the students to do it, so pay attention. Tomorrow we will have new patients, and it will be your turn." Dr. Meyer signaled to us that we should take notes, and the three of us opened our notebooks and uncapped our pens. In that much at least we were practiced. The nurse returned with Mr. Rodgers, a burly, light-skinned black man around forty. He moved slowly, and his face was tearstained. He took a seat at the table as the nurse locked the chart room door behind him.

"Mr. Rodgers, I am Dr. Begum. I will be your psychiatrist while you are here. The other people at the table are your treatment team. We will all work together to figure out how to best help you. They will introduce themselves." We went around the table and told Mr. Rodgers our names and our titles. Nurse. Social worker. Psychologist in training. He nodded through each introduction before Dr. Begum launched into his interview. "Mr. Rodgers, please tell us what brings you here."

"Sexual problems," Mr. Rodgers said in a voice that was surprisingly childish given the manly body it came from. He began to cry. Miss Smith handed him a box of tissues and he took a few. His grief was as palpable as his answer was incomplete.

"You are very upset," said Dr. Begum. "But I'd like you to try to say more so that we can understand and help you."

"When I was eight, I started to have irresistible urges. I took a nap with my mother, and I touched her inappropriately while she was sleeping." He continued to cry as he spoke. I did not want him to go on, but he did. "I've always had these urges in me. I tried to deal with them. I went to church. I prayed on it. But the urges were bigger than me. I had them toward my stepdaughter, and I couldn't help myself. She's twelve. I was alone with her too much, and finally I took her in the back room and I touched her, inappropriately. I did it a few times. I couldn't help myself. She told her teacher, and my wife kicked me out, and now there are legal proceedings. In Pennsylvania." He stopped speaking here and wept for his misfortune. I didn't doubt that he had been very unfortunate in myriad ways that he had not—and could not have—elaborated, but the twelve-year-old girl stuck in my mind. There were silence and something like repulsion around the table. "I came here to get help with my urges," he said, wiping his face and looking at us.

"Okay, we will try to help you with that," said Dr. Begum, nodding and taking notes. He went on with the assessment: How was the patient's appetite, his sleep, his interest in activities he typically found pleasurable? His interview was similar to T.'s but stiffer, hewing closely to what I'd come to understand were the *DSM*'s main differentials. T. always seemed to be trying to know the patient. Dr. Begum had more quantitative concerns. For how many weeks had the patient's appetite been poor? For what number of days had he been feeling depressed? The answers would allow us to distinguish among the manual's different mood disorders—dysthymia and major depression and depressive disorder not otherwise specified.

Adjusting my thinking to this framework had become for me like learning a foreign dialect of a familiar language. It also felt reductive. In whose reality were anyone's problems so finite and circumscribed? How many times had Mr. Rodgers's mother sanctioned their incest? How strong was his impulse to abuse his stepdaughter, on a scale from one to ten? For a psychologist the real work began after this kind of checklist conclusion; for modern psychiatry it was more or less where it ended. Dr. Begum seemed like a good doctor, thoughtful and bright and with higher expectations for his staff than they'd been able to maintain for themselves. I both admired his rigor and wondered how he maintained it—how any of them did—given the banality of his task. Arrive at diagnosis; prescribe pill. Repeat, repeat, repeat.

Mr. Rodgers was not suicidal or homicidal, he had been feeling depressed for some months, he was sleeping okay but did not have much of an appetite, he did not take real pleasure in anything lately, he was irritable, he was occasionally hearing a woman's voice telling him to kill himself, but he was not compelled to obey her. No history of substance abuse, though sometimes he'd have a drink when the woman's voice became intolerable. No previous psychiatric hospitalizations. No health problems. He had been born at Kings County Hospital, and though he now lived far away, he had last week decided to return here, as if to Mother, for help. When the interview was over, the nurse unlocked the door and let Mr. Rodgers out of our room.

"Depression with psychotic features," Dr. Begum concluded. "Who would like to follow this case?" He looked at Tamar, Bruce, and me. Were we the only therapists on the unit? I'd gathered that the social workers did discharge planning and not therapy. I wasn't sure if Dr. Meyer actually saw patients in addition to supervising. The interns who'd been there before us had spoken about the medical students who were often rotating through and also saw patients. But the others had never clarified what happened when no trainees were around at all. Would there actually be no psychotherapy whatsoever if Bruce and Tamar and I weren't there? This was not out of line with the medical model, which asserted that abnormal behavior results from physical problems and should be treated with medicine, but even at a hospital it seemed like an extreme position.

"I already have five in my caseload," said Bruce.

"I do, too," said Tamar.

And so by default I had my fourth patient. The meeting started to break up. I stayed in my seat and wondered how best to be a therapist to someone whose actions repulsed me. Dr. Meyer and Dr. Winkler stayed, too.

Dr. Meyer advised, "You need to explore his legal situation. Is he malingering to avoid his charges, or does he really have a treatable psychiatric problem? Get his permission to call his wife."

Dr. Winkler offered, "Wilhelm Reich had a similar history." Reich was one of the early and more controversial psychoanalysts, a contemporary of Freud's. "He was overstimulated as a young boy—saw some of the servants in his house doing it. Climbed into bed with his nanny when he was just a kid and started touching her. She let him. Anyway, he used his experiences to develop some interesting ideas. Track the voice Mr. Rodgers is hearing. You'll know he's getting better as it starts to become more benign."

Mr. Rumbert was still not talking, but he was no longer wrapped in a sheet, and he was willing to write. On George's inpatient unit, psychologists had dedicated rooms in which to do therapy. In the G Building, privacy was one more unattainable luxury, and we only had the dayroom with its big public space. Mr. Rumbert and I faced each other across a dining table. Around us other patients sat silently, maybe just staring or watching TV. Mornings were often quiet, before boredom got the better of people and the ruckuses began. Dressed in a crisply ironed pajama set that appeared brand-new and expensive, with erect posture and the smoothest skin, Mr. Rumbert looked regal in the sunlight, the king of Kings County. "Why am I being held here against my will?" he scribbled in my notebook. It felt odd to respond verbally, but writing back didn't seem quite right either. *I* wasn't selectively mute.

"You've been confused. You weren't taking care of yourself. You stopped eating," I said. Be specific, T. had directed.

"I'm fine," he wrote. He let me read that and then continued. "In this blessed land of America we have rights none of which have been given to me. You trap me here. I have no name tag. You pump me full of drugs, you and your Dr. T. Where's my mother?"

"She's still in New York. She'll be visiting. I'm not sure when. You can call her," I said, though of course that would be impractical as long as he refused to speak. "Or I can," I added.

"I'm still waiting for you to tell me what's wrong with me, Doctor. What!" he wrote. I felt a moment's thrill in being called doctor, even on paper, but then became unnerved by Mr. Rumbert's airs and his assertions. I knew his diagnosis, but what was he to do with the news that what was wrong with him was schizophrenia, catatonic type? And also his paranoia was contagious: *How did I really know there was anything wrong with him?* Maybe somehow his behavior made sense—his fasting and his silence and his fear that I might zap him with my eyes.

I tried a line of Dr. T.'s. "Your thoughts have gotten all mixed up," I said.

He became apoplectic, his mouth falling open, his eyes growing wide. He clearly wanted to exclaim, but he had sworn himself to silence. It was a real bind. He finally settled for raising his hands toward the ceiling, shaking them, and looked up as if to ask God to save him from my inanity. He came back down to the paper and scribbled furiously: "What? I never said my thoughts were mixed up! Never!" He looked at me imperiously before putting down my pen and padding off in his bright white socks and his pajamas.

I went to find Hong Hanh. She was in her red sweatpants sitting cross-legged on her bed, as rumpled as Mr. Rumbert was pressed.

"Good morning, Miss Hanh," I said. "Will you come with me to the dayroom to talk?" I wasn't sure how we would accomplish a conversation, but we were supposed to do at least twenty minutes of therapy a few times a week with our individual patients, and I had resolved to try despite the obvious barrier. She got up and followed me, and we took seats at a table. "I'd like to get to know you," I said to her. She looked at me.

"You tell Dr. Win-kler I no need be here?" she asked. I nodded. I had. She continued, "And no need medication. I no want medication." She was on one antipsychotic or another. Everyone there was.

"Okay," I said. "I'll tell him that, too."

We sat looking at each other. Was there nothing else to say? "Dr. Winkler suggested I ask if we could call your brother," I said. "Maybe he can help us understand—"

Miss Hanh jumped up from her chair. "No call brother. No. No," she said. She was shaking her head emphatically.

"Okay," I said, putting out my hand to signal she should sit back down and collect herself. "No call brother. Don't worry. I won't call your brother."

She sat back down. I smiled at her, and she smiled back. "You have some problems with your brother?" I asked gently.

"No call brother," she said. "No medication. I no need medication. You tell Dr. Win-kler. No medication." She stood up. Maybe this was a test. If I relayed her messages faithfully to Dr. Winkler, possibly she would begin to trust me, and that would be the beginning of a beautiful relationship. I would just have to become fluent in Vietnamese first. Hong Hanh walked off back toward her room, and I found Gabriel, which was easy because she had not left her spot by the door. I approached her.

"How are you today, Gabriel?" I asked, pulling up a chair to sit down next to her.

She answered too loudly. "I'm good," she said. "I'm just thinking, thinking and thoughting. Drinking my coffee, my caffeine, my java." I knew from my time in CPEP that her slightly odd way of talking was evidence of a thought disorder, one of the hallmarks of both schizophrenia and mania. I was relieved to identify a symptom of a genuine psychiatric problem, even if she was mostly in the G Building because she had nowhere else to go.

"You're waiting to leave for Kingsboro?" I asked.

"I am," she said, looking down her nose at me with some suspicion.

"You told me that yesterday, that's how I know," I explained.

"Well then, why are you asking again?" Her voice was always a decibel too loud.

"Just trying to make conversation," I said. She looked back toward the door. "How did you sleep last night?"

"I slept fine."

"How's your appetite?" When in doubt, I figured, ask questions about symptoms. They were so impersonal they might not scare her off.

"You're a nosy one, aren't you?" asked Gabriel.

"I'm doing a not very good job of trying to get to know you," I said. Maybe she would respond to self-deprecation.

"You can try, but I'm not going to get too close," she warned, turning her back and ending our talk.

When I met Dr. Meyer in his office for our first individual supervision, he called Gabriel "blissfully psychotic," by which I figured he meant that if your life sucked as much as hers did, you were better off being a little bit out of it. He contrasted her with Mr. Rumbert. "There are two emotional states underlying schizophrenia: terror and rage. Figure out where Mr. Rumbert is at any given moment, and help him connect those upsetting feelings to what's going on in his life," he said. "You're on his side. Let him feel that. When he asks you to tell him what's wrong with him, be as concrete as possible. Remind him again, 'You stopped eating and speaking. Those are signs that something's not going right.' See where he takes it from there." He said that I could communicate my support to Hong Hanh, too, despite the language barrier. "Look, obviously the situation is not ideal, but you can help her to feel better cared for here just by checking in with her every day. Hopefully, she'll be your first and last non-English-speaking patient, but she won't be the only one who thinks she doesn't need to be here. The first thing to work on with someone like Hong is what went wrong that led to the hospitalization. Until a patient can take in the fact that there is a problem, there can't be any treatment."

If the Mafia is out to kidnap you, a locked inpatient unit is a great place to hide out, but try convincing a paranoid woman that she's safe there. "I want my mother contacted when they take me," the patient, a Ms. Anders, was declaring loudly and angrily to the treatment team as I took a seat in the morning meeting. I was late because, upstairs, Scott Brent had seen Bruce and me laughing in the hallway and had asked us suspiciously what was going on. Nothing was going on. Caitlin watched the whole interaction from her doorjamb, and when Scott had gone into his office and closed the door, she explained that it was his birthday and that he believed the interns were planning something for him. When we told her that we hadn't known, and further that we had no plans, she told us that we'd better make some. Bruce and I went into our own office, and I shut the door. Bruce declared, "Oh, good Lord!" which I thought summed things up nicely.

As a group, we interns had months ago identified that Scott had a narcissistic character style. If depressives feel guilty and bad, narcissists feel empty and inferior. Their fragile self-esteem requires constant shoring up. They don't easily let go of perceived snubs like not being allowed to handpick all the interns or not having their every decision applauded, their every birthday marked. I hadn't spent four years in a doctoral program in psychology not to know how to placate a narcissist, but the very idea of having to do it exhausted me. Besides, it was a cynical task, this avoidance of slighting him, and I preferred to maintain the belief that Scott was better than that, closer to what I needed him to be, even though there was nothing but my wishing to support this. I told Bruce I couldn't work up the energy to care about Caitlin's dramatics and didn't think that he should either. Instead, feeling burdened, he tracked down Alisa, the most sympathetic of our intern group, and the two of them went to troll East Flatbush for a cake. When I arrived late to the morning meeting, the treatment team, save for Dr. Meyer, was assembled, and Dr. Winkler was gently questioning Ms. Anders, all eyes on her.

"Usually, people kidnap for money. Do you have a lot of money?" he asked.

"No," she replied, hostility in her voice.

"So why do they want to kidnap you?"

"Hate. They hate me."

"Are you hearing voices?" he asked.

"This is New York City. There are people talking around me all the time. How would I know if they were just voices?"

"You plug your ears," he told her. "If the voices you're hearing don't get quieter, they're coming from inside your head, and you'll know you're hallucinating."

"You're not paying attention," she told Dr. Winkler. "Everyone here knows I'm going to be kidnapped by the Mafia!"

"No, they don't," he said matter-of-factly. Dr. Winkler was the only person I'd ever heard speak to the most chronic psychiatric inpatients as if they were fully human, without condescension or pity or something worse. "Is there anything in your life you're feeling guilty about?"

"No," she said. "I have no traffic tickets. I haven't killed anyone."

"Did you ever want to kill anyone?"

"Are we done here?" she asked haughtily, standing up.

"Sure, for now," Dr. Winkler said, nodding toward one of the social workers, who unlocked the door to let Ms. Anders return to her room to await her fate.

"Paranoid delusions are preceded by a sense of guilt over some long-ago event that's been obscured over time, and delusions about the Mafia are very common," Dr. Winkler told Tamar and me and the two medical students, Steve and Jason, who had joined us on the unit that week. "We need to bring the family in to provide a realistic correction to her fear that they're in danger. They come in and challenge her thinking, unhinge the whole delusional system. Who wants to follow Ms. Anders's case?" he asked, and Tamar volunteered.

As another new patient was located outside, Dr. Begum told Tamar and me that one of us would lead the next evaluation. Tamar nodded in assent, and I felt relieved. The little old Caribbean man who was brought in answered her questions about his symptoms and his history succinctly. He was as psychotic as any other patient, but he obviously knew his way around a psychiatric screening. When Tamar had finished, Dr. Begum asked if he had any questions for the team. The patient paused and thought and then asked: "Do American women like to have sex in bed?"

Dr. Begum replied, "Yes, I hear that they do," and then we all got up from the table to leave. I walked down the hallway to Mr. Rumbert's room. He'd started speaking aloud again the day before, which turned out to be more trying than his silence.

"How do you *know* that's my name?" he asked when I addressed him by his name.

"How do you *know* my mother came to see me yesterday?" he asked when I inquired about the woman's visit. It was like trying to talk to a freshman philosophy major who'd just watched the entire *Matrix* trilogy. When I offered him the chance to correct any misinformation I might have, he became indignant and announced that he wasn't going to speak again until discharge. I told him this would make it difficult for us to let him go, as T. had taught me to say to ER patients who didn't want to cooperate.

"Are you threatening me?" he asked. I wasn't quite,

though I could see why he saw it that way. The next day we met with his mother and Dr. Winkler in the dayroom. It was my first family meeting on inpatient. Families could play an important role in recovery—or sabotage it altogether—but so far none of my other patients had relatives interested in showing up. I got Mr. Rumbert from his room, and he followed after me in his socks. When we sat down at a table still jelly stained from breakfast, Dr. Winkler asked how he was doing.

"I've been thinking a lot about what I am and how people see me," he said.

"'Oh would some power the gift to give us, to see ourselves as others see us!'" replied Dr. Winkler. "Robert Burns."

Mr. Rumbert explained that this was especially on his mind because he was having trouble with his vision. He couldn't see himself clearly, and he couldn't tell if he was eating the right things, "what the Bible says you should eat."

"Does the Bible tell you to starve yourself to death?" asked Dr. Winkler. Mr. Rumbert shook his head, and Dr. Winkler went on. "The Bible says many things, lots of them contradictory." They discussed some of these. Mr. Rumbert's mother asked when she could take her son home to Barbados. "We have to figure out what medicines work for him and then work out a treatment plan for after discharge," Dr. Winkler told her.

"How do I know when a medicine is working for me?" asked Mr. Rumbert.

"What works is what helps you eat, sleep, and concentrate," Dr. Winkler explained.

The next day Mr. Rumbert was as open with me as he'd been. "Am I clean?" he asked when I greeted him. He sounded worried. He explained that his problem with his sight left him unable to tell. I told him he looked quite clean to me and asked him what it meant to him to be dirty. "That no human would want to get near me," he replied.

"What would happen then?" I asked and then heard Dr. T. in my head: "Too complicated."

"Bizarre ideation," Dr. Winkler labeled Mr. Rumbert's thinking when we spoke. Psychotic symptoms had delightful names. They rolled off the tongue. Flight of ideas. Phonemic paraphasias. "How's it going with Mr. Rodgers?" he asked.

The child molester. I was seeing him three times a week, as I was expected to, and tolerating it by learning about his history and avoiding his present. This probably wasn't the way to go. It was no kind of telescopic lens. He told me he'd married an older woman soon after graduating high school, and then had four children with her. She had an affair and he left. After one year as a single man he'd married again—the woman with the daughter. He tried to solve the problem of his untoward sexual desires in church. It hadn't worked. He remained pretty depressed, I told Dr. Winkler—though the voice endorsing suicide had faded as the antipsychotic medication took effect and he remained outside the jurisdiction of the Pennsylvania police. We could begin to think about discharging him. Mr. Rodgers's father had called to say that he would take his son home within a few days to face his legal troubles with his stepdaughter. I would talk to Mr. Rodgers about how he wanted to proceed with his charges. Would he plead out? Go to trial? What were the likely outcomes of each? It wasn't therapy, but it was all that I could stomach, and maybe it would even be marginally useful to him.

- - - - - - - - -

There was a twenty-five-year-old deaf and mute patient on the unit. Her name was Camara. One night she apparently fainted and fell, and the next morning a roly-poly white man none of us had ever seen before appeared at our meeting, identifying himself as a clinical case manager and suggesting that the chart note indicate that Camara had "placed herself on the floor." I tried to make eye contact with someone on the team to confirm that this was lunacy, but no one met my gaze. Apparently, the word "fall" did not go lightly into a chart. The fainting had been no one's fault, and Camara had not hurt herself, but every patient was a legal proceeding waiting to happen, every staff member a potential accused assailant. As if the patients' paranoia were not enough to leave the fifth floor bursting at its cracking seams, the staff's almost matched it most weeks. The Justice Department's impending arrival only inflamed this, and we were reminded of it in one way or another daily. (By the constant painting and repainting of the first floor, for one: Did DOJ prefer teal to aquamarine? The question was obviously keeping somebody up nights.) The atmosphere on the unit was so fraught that I could almost feel sympathy for the somber and silent recreation therapist who locked himself alone in the cavernous group room from nine to five each day. If you didn't interact with anyone, there was less to worry about. But then there was the fact that there were no groups being run on the unit, and that even the interns' pleas to use the space—*which did not after all technically belong to this man*—to run therapy groups for a couple of hours a week had gone unanswered. (Actually, he nodded when Bruce and I asked to use the room, but then he disappeared at the agreed-upon time, along with the room's only key.) Was a "group" one burned-out city employee hiding alone for hours in "the group room"? The answer, it seemed, was yes. In contrast, in casual conversation George would occasionally launch into a story with a line like, "One of my inpatients left knitting group today to go check her e-mail . . . ," and my mouth would fall open. *Knitting group? E-mail?* The next day I would report on the bounties of the private hospital to my fellow Kings County interns, who would gather like orphans around Annie just back from Daddy Warbucks's to hear my dispatches. What puzzled me almost as much as the recreation therapist's blatant shirking of his sole responsibility was that he went by the title "Doctor," even though he was not one.

Still, "Dr." Jacobs's behavior made other things on G–51 seem less weird in comparison. Like: members of the treatment team sometimes addressed floridly psychotic patients with frustration and cries of "You're not making any sense!" (Not making any sense was exactly why they were in our company, so yelling at them for it seemed particularly unreasonable.) Like: Dr. Meyer rarely showed his face on the unit after the interns' first week there, and no one seemed to find his absence even worth mentioning.

The last point got to me. Dr. Meyer was the one psychologist assigned to the unit, and from what I could tell, he almost never actually set foot on the unit. I met with him in his office once a week for forty-five minutes of individual supervision, and when he wasn't reminding me to carve out a place for my field with my notes—refer to voices as "auditory hallucinations," to alcohol as "EtOH"—he was helpful and engaging. For example, when I shared with him my strategy for helping a psychotic patient manage his feelings about having been abused as a child—"Try not to think about it," I told him—Dr. Meyer diplomatically replied, "That's one way to go." I explained that while I would never suggest such a thing to an outpatient, on inpatient I was trying to prepare the man for discharge by building his defenses.

"Which defense is that?" he'd asked.

"Repression," I said.

"Defenses operate unconsciously," he reminded me. "This is obviously already on his mind. Ask him why he's thinking about his abuse now."

What I was thinking about as I sat with Dr. Meyer, as the weeks went by, was this: Did we psychologists matter at all here? In the ER, T. ruled her own little world. Unencumbered by anyone or anything, she made use of her space to be a psychologist, to be always planting seeds. On inpatient, larger forces seemed to have come together to silently assert psychology's insignificance. All the trainees who came onto G-51 were treated equally, no matter their training or experience. The interns were appreciated as extra bodies who could give the patients attention, but never as if our specific knowledge of psychological functioning was of any particular value. And so Jason, the dentist training to be an oral surgeon and doing his mandatory ten-day psychiatric rotation, had as many patients as I did, but with less supervision (I wasn't sure he had any, actually). Had he learned, as I had, that paranoia is the externalization of one's own aggressive impulses? That delusions represent the unconscious wishes of the parents? That auditory hallucinations result from the projection of the pathological introject of the mother? Did he even know what an introject was? Granted, I had little experience in actually treating the sickest people, but I had at least spent many years in school learning how to think about human health and pathology. That seemed of little repute here. Dr. Begum was always making noise about getting the staff in order, but he left Dr. Meyer out of this equation. If he believed that psychology had something to contribute to his unit, wouldn't he remark upon my recalcitrant supervisor? It wasn't clear that anyone other than Tamar and Bruce and me took note of Dr. Meyer's absence, or even whether the chain of command would entitle anyone to say anything if they did. Maybe it wasn't Dr. Begum's place to remind Dr. Meyer to show up. I didn't know. All I did know was that everyone who worked there seemed to have a sense of his or her own distinct purpose and that my supervisor's actions communicated that at the very least he himself felt his—and by extension likely ours—not worthy of fulfilling.

Dr. Begum went away on vacation, and Dr. Winkler was left to manage everyone on his own, but having been around forever, he was either less concerned about getting the staff to behave themselves or less self-defeating. Attendance at the morning meeting became sparse—none of the nurses, none of the social workers. Tamar left to do her month with Dr. T. in CPEP, and Bruce—whose already thin patience with the hospital had dissolved completely after a few weeks of morning meetings—avoided the fifth floor as much as possible. So much for my longed-for camaraderie. I sat in the chart room with Jason and Steve, the medical students. The two had settled in comfortably and quickly. Jason was the dentist. Steve was young, skinny, eager—the first medical student I'd met to date who actually wanted to become a psychiatrist. They were likable enough, but I found their self-assurance abrasive, so certain did they seem that completing any kind of medical training somehow qualified them to be working with crazy people. That I'd studied the human mind all those years and still imagined myself grossly unprepared stood out against their contented certitude, and I briefly wondered whose distortion was more problematic.

"Who wants a new patient, a Mr. Bernard?" asked Dr. Winkler, beginning the meeting.

"I do," I said. "The ones I have are mostly disposition problems at this point." Which meant that they were only on the unit because they had nowhere else to go, and also that I had given up on them, just like everyone else before me. I was talking about Hong Hanh and Gabriel. Mr. Rumbert—stabilized, I guessed, by an antipsychotic medication—had started talking and eating regularly, and so had gone home with his mother. Mr. Rodgers had taken as much of a break as he could from his miserable family/legal situation and was about to leave as well. The day before, I'd said good-bye to a Mr. Mower, who had emerged from the deepest ebb of his depression nicely with meds or time or conversation and whose departure I'd figured out how to expedite myself when no one else was willing to go downstairs to the pharmacy to fill his prescription in time for him to leave that day.

Steve turned to Jason: "Do you want Mr. Bernard?"

Jason to Steve: "Do you?"

"I'll take him," said Steve, making his announcement to Dr. Winkler. It was as if I had not spoken at all.

"Sure, never mind me," I said with more resentment than I cared to show, but still considerably less than I felt. They seemed to consider me, a mere psychologist, no more than a planet—a moon—to their sun.

Steve and Jason were all apologies, and I had a new patient.

Dr. Winkler went to retrieve Mr. Bernard from the hallway. He was in his seventies, African American with drooping eyelids and age spots, too thin, and barely able to walk in a straight line. Dr. Winkler helped him into a chair. Could he possibly be drunk or high after having spent at least the last twenty-four hours in G-ER?

"Do you know where you are, Mr. Bernard?" asked Dr. Winkler, skimming the chart as he began the interview. If he couldn't answer that first crucial question, our assessment would be brief, and I would resort to calling his family to learn about him, if there was any family to call.

"Is this the projects?" guessed Mr. Bernard, his pink tongue and globules of spittle entering the space in his mouth where his bottom teeth were once rooted in better times.

"Do you know how you've spent the last couple of days?" Dr. Winkler asked, reframing his first question.

Mr. Bernard paused to reflect. "I've been in meetings and consultations with the governor."

Jason and Steve tried to hide their smirks. Mr. Bernard's psychosis, whether substance induced or otherwise, did not make him a good therapy case. My indignation had won me no prize.

"Do you have any medical problems?" asked Dr. Winkler.

Mr. Bernard thought and then told us, "I don't have a heart."

"What was that?" asked Dr. Winkler. His hearing wasn't great.

"He doesn't have a heart," I said loudly.

"Oh. How is that?" asked Dr. Winkler.

"My old lady ate it!" replied my new patient, outraged.

Steve and Jason could barely hold their laughter until Mr. Bernard was out of the room. "You guys want to thank me for taking this one?" I asked, and they nodded and continued to chuckle.

Dr. Winkler looked at us with a serious face: " 'An insane man forsakes reason and often speaks the truth. A sane man holds his tongue.' Henry Miller. Just because someone's psychotic doesn't mean he isn't telling the truth." Steve and Jason stopped their laughing.

Dr. Winkler looked back in Mr. Bernard's chart and found

his daughter's number. "Call her," he instructed me. "Find out how many years he's been drinking. Could be Korsakoff's dementia. Alcoholics get it from chronic thiamine deficiency. This is a good case. Interesting," he said, nodding to me on his way out of the chart room. I reached for the chart and the phone.

Mr. Bernard's daughter was exasperated but helpful. "He's been a drunk his whole adult life," she told me. "He finished a two-year inpatient rehab about six months ago and had been sober as far as I could tell since. But a couple of weeks ago he started complaining that one of his neighbors was bothering him, and he had that irritable tone. I figured he'd started with the drinking again. I gave up on trying to save him a long time ago and haven't talked to him since the complaining started. I'm self-protective at this point. Did his neighbor bring him in?"

Consulting the chart, I affirmed this. She asked with a sigh, "When are visiting hours?"

With so many people from so many different nations both working and residing on the unit, the details of conversations were sometimes lost, and sometimes hard-won. For example, when an obese manic woman spoke, during her initial interview, of the dildo her son had recently purchased for her, Dr. Begum had to stop the proceedings to clarify what that was. The morning meeting was hardly a delicate environment, but still no one rushed to offer an explanation.

Sometimes it was less vocabulary and more pronunciation that was a stumbling block. When Dr. Begum returned to New York from what felt to me like a very long vacation, I sat in as he interviewed an immigrant from Africa. Her answers to his questions were just vague enough to be bizarre, which was of course diagnostic. "Tell us why you are here?" he began in his Bangladeshi clip.

"I came here to rest," the young woman, whose name was Mpenzi, said. She wore a colorful turban around her hair. Her Kenyan accent was melodious to my ear.

"How old are you?" he asked.

"Twentysomething," she replied, smiling beatifically. "You'd have to ask my mother."

"How is your mother doing?" he inquired, because family history, and especially of mental illness, which runs in families, was always important.

"She's fine. Doing well," said Mpenzi.

"Where does she live?" asked Dr. Begum, who would want us to get the woman in, or at least on the phone, ASAP.

"She's in heaven," replied the patient.

Dr. Begum turned to me, his de facto American sidekick: "Is that in New Jersey?"

Mpenzi became my patient. It turned out that she was a permanent resident of Kingsboro, sent to us after a manic episode for stabilization, though she must have mostly achieved as much in the ER because she was placid for the week that I knew her, her most pronounced symptom a long-standing and exciting delusion that Kanye West was on his way to New York to marry her. She hoped to be back at Kingsboro before the Christmas holiday for a party that was apparently not to be missed.

I could not avoid doing inpatient interviews in front of the team forever, and finally Dr. Begum instructed me to lead one. Dr. Winkler was sensitive and encouraging. "This is like dentistry," he said to me as we waited for our new charge to be brought in. "You have to get the patient to open up."

Her name was Ivory. She was pregnant and addicted to crack. She stared into the distance instead of looking at me and complained that she was not getting any good snacks. I ran through the points of focus I'd written in my notebook— presenting problem, history of the presenting problem, psychiatric history, family history, health problems, drug use, forensic history. She answered me but was so depressed that I quickly began feeling hopeless myself and missed some things. It wasn't the end of the world. Dr. Begum stepped in to fill in the blanks, and I took in what I'd missed, the information that would help us arrive at the diagnosis. (Substance-induced depression—you couldn't diagnose anything but substance-induced fill-in-the-blank as long as the patient had recently used.) "Good job," Dr. Begum said after, smiling as he always did. "Each time you'll get a little better."

And if "better" meant "more comfortable," I did, just a few days later with a patient named Garrett Miller who had checked himself in for homicidal thinking. He was a few years sober, depressed, and hearing voices. Major depressive disorder, severe, with psychotic features. When I told Dr. Meyer about him in supervision, he wasn't buying it. "In the winter one in four psychiatric patients are malingering," he told me. It was December.

I liked working with Garrett, though. He was a talker, coherent, and with the typically tragic story. His father had been killed when he was two, shot to death through an apartment door he was pounding on, by an elderly neighbor who'd asked him to bring her some groceries. Garrett's own homicidal fantasies had been directed toward the wife of his closest cousin. "She was annoying me," he said, which seemed like a thin motive for murderous thoughts. Garrett's cousin had just gotten out of jail, and the wife was being possessive of his time. "I was there for him for four years while he was locked up. Where was she?" he wanted to know.

I said he seemed to have a lot of anger toward women.

"I was raised by women," he protested, as if that would invalidate my observation. "Everyone here is so fucked up," he complained to me. "I feel like I have to take care of them all." That was something to note.

"You're always taking care of people, but you never feel you get any care in return," I observed. For the first time he agreed with me, but he did not want to say more. "My life is half over anyway." He was only thirty-six. "What does it matter?" he asked. Often, on inpatient, there was a certain and predictable shutting down. Even when cognitively capable of it, no one on G-51 wanted to think too closely about himself. This was a large part of the problem.

Garrett was one more patient who couldn't leave because he didn't have anywhere else to go. The G Building was not supposed to discharge people to the homeless shelters, as this was either inhumane or a surefire route to a quick readmission. The social workers were kept incredibly busy finding state-sponsored housing programs for those who were functionally homeless, but both Oswald and Miss Smith had disappeared, so no one was working toward Garrett's departure. He was a voluntary patient and was perfectly happy to stay, which made me think that perhaps Dr. Meyer had been right to suspect that he'd been malingering the voices and the homicidal thoughts. You could choose to see this as sociopathic or incredibly resourceful: once a patient was admitted to G, a team of people went to work on the case, in the end providing a reasonable place to live if nothing more. Most days I admired Garrett's ingenuity, though I was being at least tacitly lied to in the process, which also made me resentful. Still, in the wake of the mysterious disappearance of the social workers (why did no one on the unit bother to tell anyone else when they were planning lengthy absences?), I took it upon myself, with a martyr's attitude, to get a name of a housing program for recovering drug addicts and to start the process of applying to it for him. That wasn't my job, but I didn't want him to end up like Gabriel or Hong Hanh or the patient who had been the talk of the building days earlier when she finally left for Kingsboro after an entire decade on the fourth floor of G.

Garrett and I had been working together for a few weeks when I came in one morning to find him enraged. Camara, the deaf and mute patient, had accused a few of the men on the unit of sexually assaulting her late in the night, and Garrett was one of them. He couldn't tolerate that anyone would think he was capable of such a thing. I took in his indignation and felt apologetic on behalf of the staff. Later I spoke to Dr. Winkler about the whole thing. "She went to one of the night nurses right after," he told me. "The doctor on call came up and did a sniff test of all the men's hands. Garrett tested positive." Camara was transferred to another unit. Maybe her family was going to press charges.

I was so pissed off at Garrett that I didn't want to work with him anymore, which was probably understandable and definitely unacceptable. He was assigned to me no matter what, and it was my job to understand and work through my feelings in order to function as his therapist. This was an absolute. "Whoever walks into your office is your patient," Dr. Aronoff had once said to me pointedly. She meant: no matter what, you can't act on your feelings with people who have come to see you in good faith. Acting on feelings was what people did *outside* the consulting room, and it was what made the therapeutic relationship different from all others. It involved the therapist thinking in place of reacting, maybe the most crucial part of a treatment. I needed to be curious about what Garrett was up to: What kind of reaction was he unconsciously intent upon stimulating with his behavior? How could the treatment team use this information to help him know himself better? If I abandoned him in rage and disgust, that was hardly of any use to him, and being of use to him was why I was there, even if no one else managed to see it that way.

But two months on G-51 had worn me down. I was cranky. No one else on the unit bothered to rein in the feelings patients evoked in them—or even probably to consider them—so why should I? I certainly wasn't getting much encouragement. Dr. Meyer had recently gone completely MIA along with the social workers. Helpful as Dr. Begum and Dr. Winkler were on the fly, they were too busy to sit down for a discussion of any length. Dr. Begum at least—contemporary, symptom-focused psychiatrist that he was—was unlikely to be able to provide the kind of teaching I was looking for anyway, not that he didn't wish it were otherwise. (He had recently gleefully announced to me that he was a patient in psychoanalysis himself and that "this depth psychology is so much more interesting than the pills!") The unit was clearly lacking in psychological mindedness—an appreciation of the value of reflecting on one's own psychology. This was its weak point.

As Marvin Mavin and patients like him had continued to terrorize the fifth floor, no one talked about what they were acting out or how the treatment team was failing to help them contain their aggression; they just restrained them and shot them full of Haldol. This was not done malevolently; it seemed to someone the best way to keep them from harming themselves and others. But it only worked until the next time, which without any *psychological* treatment was sure to come, and it left the other patients feeling unsafe besides. "If I had a grenade, there'd be no people like that left on earth," Gabriel had said to me, with clenched fists, one morning after Marvin had lurched threateningly around the dayroom while she and I sat together. Her hands and voice shook as she spoke. She was increasingly disorganized for the rest of that day.

It was an imperfect unit in an imperfect system, and sometimes the clamoring hopelessness made it hard to hear yourself think. For too many reasons to count, this thing had developed in the G Building, this culture of offhand neglect. No one inside quite escaped it: certainly not the patients, and then, too, not the interns. But I had the resources to surmount it, if only for myself. "Graduate school teaches you how to teach yourself," a professor of mine had said toward the end. I left Gabriel that day to go home and order a book on psychological treatment in inpatient settings. I paid extra for expedited shipping. The text arrived with the first snowfall just as I officially lost my supervisor. Dr. Meyer, who'd apparently been out of town interviewing and otherwise using his sick time to stay as far from G as he possibly could, finally gave his two weeks' notice, suburban outpatient clinic bound. "This is no place to spend ten years," he cautioned Tamar and Bruce and me as we clustered in his office to watch him pack his books. I didn't aspire to any kind of drawn-out stay, but I wanted to get something out of the two months I had left on G-51. I went home and started reading.

CHAPTER SEVEN

MY NEW BOOK KEPT ME GOOD COMPANY, LIKE THE VOLLEY-
ball Wilson to Tom Hanks's castaway. *Of course psychological
treatment is important for psychological problems*, it told me. *Here
is how psychologists have an impact on inpatient wards*, it went on.
This had much to do with what I suspected: conveying that
"symptoms" were more than just arbitrary neurological events;
encouraging the team to be thoughtful about their own emotional reactions; talking to patients individually and in groups
to help them make sense of their experiences and concerns.
I carried the scholarly tome with me each morning to read
on the subway. That it did not prove a corrective to the low
professional self-esteem that I had been blaming on my environment was my first clue—well, maybe not my first—that
my actual problem was more of an internally generated one.
It covered familiar ground, this heightened attention I paid to
voices I heard as disparaging. But I could know this for only a
moment before I'd forget it again and do the whole thing over.

The irritable mood that grew out of this conundrum was

not winning me any popularity contests on the sixth floor, as I shuffled between Caitlin's office and Scott's. The two of them were always around up on six. They were the white noise of our days. For months I'd been enraged, if unfairly, with Caitlin, for offering what I knew passed as therapy supervision at a hospital, but was nowhere near as good as what I had gotten used to in grad school. I retaliated most weeks during our time together by using all the theoretical language I could muster (and I'd learned quite a bit of it) to make Caitlin feel dumb—her Achilles' heel, even though she had a Ph.D. and the title of neuropsychologist. I might have felt too guilty to keep it up had she not been giving the meanness back to me in equal measure. She was a real hard-ass and a misanthrope. We went back and forth in our mutual aggression until the relationship felt like a tennis match. Sometimes I thought we were just having fun.

As for Scott, he was steadily indifferent to the charms I peacocked before him, and he bristled toward me only further when I went to him with things worth complaining about, like that my supervisors were evading me. I knew that he didn't want to hear what as our director he needed to know, but I persisted in trying to tell him, to bolster his self-esteem in this back-channel way, by demonstrating my clear expectation that he was capable of his new job—as if this might eventually both make him better at it *and* win me his love. In this I wasn't alone, as he had finally come to occupy a curious and similar place for all of us interns: we found ourselves trying to maintain fondness for him despite his oftentimes egregious unlikability. We would joke about it tenderly among ourselves when he was unresponsive to our concerns, or checked his e-mail multiple times during supervision sessions, or let us know in no uncertain terms that our careers going forward would ever be dependent on his good graces. The latter seemed to tragically illuminate his fragility. He yearned for us to feel his import and power. Us. *The interns.*

Most weeks, though, Caitlin and Scott were just low-level annoyances, and my resentment and self-doubt might have been milder had the inpatient unit been the only place I was encountering strong ambivalence about psychology. Instead, it seemed to come up everywhere I went across the hospital campus. In the face of what felt like an onslaught against my field, I had considerable difficulty holding firmly to all that I vehemently believed to be true. The more I struggled to maintain a sense of my own value, the more I wanted to lash out against an amorphous enemy.

One adversary took form in a seminar on cognitive-behavioral therapy, or CBT, where I found insult heaped not on my profession in general but on my particular psychological orientation. The main premise of CBT is that problems in living originate in cognitive and behavioral factors, which can be changed via skills learned in psychotherapy. The guiding principle of psychoanalytic therapy is that problems in living originate in the unconscious, which needs to be better understood in order to wield less influence. CBT therapists often write psychoanalytic therapy off as fantastical and impractical. Psychoanalytic clinicians tend to find CBT superficial and transiently helpful at best. CBT trainees learn how to follow treatment manuals: each session is sketched out in advance in workbooks that address particular symptoms. Psychoanalytic clinicians are trained by reading theory and case studies and seeing and discussing patients in order to learn how to think about how people function. We are also expected to be in our own therapy, not least so we can understand our emotional responses to our patients in order to use those for the good of treatment rather than for its ill. In my graduate program, if you weren't yourself in therapy, it was a fierce and unwieldy secret. In contrast, Bruce had actually been told by the director of his CBT-oriented graduate program at a respected university in Massachusetts that anyone who needed psychotherapy had no business being a doctoral student in clinical psychology.

Like many of the internships in New York City, Kings County's was psychoanalytically oriented, but because this way of thinking had been coming under fire, training programs were attempting to become "integrative." And so the interns were offered an ongoing seminar on CBT, taught by the hospital's CBT expert, Dr. Edward Levine. I tried to go in with an open mind. Dr. Levine—himself, as he told us, once the patient in a psychoanalytic therapy gone awry—had no such intention. In the first seminar, during which we were ostensibly learning about how to teach patients to relax, it was clear that we were also being indoctrinated against our preferred way of working. "A psychoanalytic stance means being quiet and listening because you don't know what else to do," Dr. Levine scoffed by way of introduction—as if this were a bad thing. He knew that most of us in the class had invested the last four years of our lives in just that sort of training, and I wasn't sure how he imagined demeaning our efforts fit in with helping us to consider alternate methods. To help myself decompress during the ninety-minute seminar that followed, I came up with the behavioral technique of making a hash mark in my notebook every time Dr. Levine insulted my orientation. By the end of the first hour, I had drawn eleven sharp vertical lines, but I didn't feel relaxed at all.

As the course wore on, Dr. Levine eventually told us more about himself, including that he was the son of Holocaust survivors. The context of this was confessional, as he went on to say that he sometimes felt undercurrents of resentment toward his traumatized patients, whenever he deemed their ordeals less horrifying than Auschwitz. This sharing of his difficulties actually softened me toward Dr. Levine, though I continued to keep a running tally each week of his derisions of my theoretical orientation. I'd counted as many as fourteen in a single ninety-minute class. Philosophical differences about what makes therapy effective aside, I also found his material as flat as the midwestern plains. If a patient was depressed, he told us, she needed to be participating in more rewarding behaviors. What kinds of things does she enjoy doing? Suggest that she do these things. Had I shown up at Dr. Aronoff's office and found this the best she had to offer, I would have given up all hope in psychotherapy forever.

As certain as I was of this, something nagged at me in CBT class, something I couldn't let go of. Dr. Levine was smart and experienced, and if he believed so resolutely that something was so, well, couldn't it be? On one hand I valued what I knew and believed, but then I would come up against this wall, the bulwark of his omniscience, his insistence that psychoanalytic treatment was bad. I couldn't quite manage to hold on to my own sense of myself in the face of this older man's certitude. It was at the heart of why I left his conference room riled up each week, rather than simply bemused by his pronounced obsession with my psychoanalytic camp, his nominal enemy.

After 9/11, Dr. Levine had worked with a handful of New York City first responders. One of his patients in particular—a fireman who'd been tasked with getting people out of the towers—had wound up especially forlorn, paralyzed by his memories, withdrawing from family and friends, and rarely leaving his house for fear that a horrible fate would befall him.

With Dr. Levine's help, over a number of months the man had become much less symptomatic. When the therapy ended, Dr. Levine asked the grateful man to come in to be filmed talking about his treatment, for teaching purposes. Dr. Levine would show us the tape to illustrate a patient's take on CBT for post-traumatic stress disorder.

The burly and upset former firefighter was painful to watch. Almost all of the interns had been in the city on that astonishing day, and the man's palpable distress took us back some years. My fellow intern Zeke left the room halfway through and didn't want to talk about it later. When the tape ended, Dr. Levine mentioned this as an aside: the patient had been wearing scrubs in the video, and this was because he had shown up on the day of its recording in his street clothes but covered in soot. "He forgot our appointment until the last minute, and he'd been doing some construction on his house. So he rushed over here like that. I had to give him something else to put on, and the scrubs were all I could get my hands on!" Dr. Levine obviously found this mildly amusing.

Not for the first time in that class, I felt discombobulated by what I was hearing, or rather by what was missing from what I was hearing. The patient, who had needed therapy in the aftermath of a trauma that resulted in becoming covered in ash, *had shown up to memorialize this treatment covered in ash.* How stubbornly attached to the denial of a dynamic unconscious did one need to be to write such an episode off as mere comical coincidence? Whether it was a focus of one's therapeutic efforts or not, its significance could not seriously be called into question, could it? And so I raised my hand. I didn't usually ask anything in that class. In the midst of all the breathing techniques and muscle relaxation exercises there seemed little worth my inquiry. "Dr. Levine," my voice wavered, "don't you find it interesting that on the day he was to be videotaped he came in looking like he did at the end of 9/11?"

Hadn't he been waiting for one of us to ask? He looked surprised by the idea. "No," he said, shrugging it off. "He just forgot."

I knew with a certainty that made the nerves at the back of my neck constrict that the ash had meaning, that the fireman had unconsciously been using it to communicate something of his experience—that despite his progress some work remained to be done. I wondered about the patient's intuitive sense of Dr. Levine's secret resentment, and about my teacher's own intolerable associations to ash. To find none of this meaningful, I guess I could understand as so much defensiveness, but I could also hardly fathom it at the same time.

So there it was: the proof I needed. Could this finally be the point where I put aside my depressive faith in my own low value? When I achieved a Zen-like comfort with all that I knew, with my orientation in particular and then, as a derivative of my newfound self-assurance, with the absolute value of psychology in general? I told the story of the ash again and again, to anyone who had enough patience to listen, but the answer I found was still no. Somehow, down deep, I was holding hard to my belief that Dr. Levine knew a deeper truth than I, simply because he said it was so. The administrators who failed to hire psychologists. Medical psychiatry. Scott Brent. Dr. Levine. I couldn't drown out the messages they delivered, and from the deepest place I couldn't let go of the certain belief that any and all of them were right.

CHAPTER EIGHT

I RETURNED TO G-51 AFTER THE WINTER HOLIDAYS TO TWO pieces of news: Gabriel had finally left for Kingsboro, and Hong's apartment—her last hope for a return to an independent life—had been sold by her legal guardian. I was sorry not to have had the chance to say good-bye to Gabriel and was rendered speechless by the kicker to the real estate proceeding, which was that every last penny of the tens of thousands of dollars Hong profited from the sale was now owed to the hospital for her protracted and involuntary stay. It was poetic injustice.

As I had learned to expect, no one on the unit knew if Hong had been told. I guessed it was my job to deliver the information, but I wasn't sure if her English covered such complicated concepts, or even if it was just better for her well-being not to know. After months of her persistent pleas, Dr. Winkler had finally agreed to take her off her meds a few weeks before, and she looked better without them. On the antipsychotics she'd suffered from akathisia, an unfortunate and common side effect that makes users restless, leaving them to pace and rock and march in place, which Hong had done, a constant jittery two-step. I still had no idea what went on in her head, which seemed an insurmountable impediment to therapy, but in her calm state she looked more and more as if she didn't need inpatient treatment anyway, and the idea that her institutionalization was some kind of horrible mistake haunted me. I both knew this couldn't be possible (there were just too many people involved in being found legally incompetent) and feared that it was so. My half delusion surely had a lot to do with Hong's own fantasies but also with the carelessness I had seen play out in my months on inpatient. Things like this happened: Hong, reluctant to let the nurses as much as take her temperature, had finally agreed that her blood could be drawn for the tests that were necessary precursors to transferring to Kingsboro. But then the blood was left to sit around for too long, and it hemolyzed, making its potassium levels appear elevated and too high for the state facility to accept her. The whole trauma of the needle had been for naught and would have to be repeated, which was nothing if not an ironic parallel to Hong's personal and political history. How could I maintain any faith in a system in which such things were as likely to happen as not?

Dr. Winkler and I talked and ultimately agreed that treating Hong with dignity meant keeping her fully informed. I went to find her, which took less time than I would've liked, given the message I didn't want to deliver. She sat on her bed in her sweatpants and her pajama top. I summoned her from the doorway, and she followed me to the dayroom, where we sat in plastic chairs and entered what had become, as the days had grown shorter and then longer again, a tentative companionable silence. "Hong," I finally began, "I have to tell you some bad news. It's about your apartment. Your guardian has sold your apartment." She jumped up from her seat.

"Tell guardian they no sell apat-ment!"

Her feet were firmly planted. Her arms hung in the air as if in suspended animation while she waited for my reply.

"I can't, Hong, it's already done. They sold it. The apartment is gone."

"Tell guardian they no sell apat-ment!" she insisted. Again I tried to explain, and again she failed to understand, or to accept—who knew. I hadn't even told her the worst part. *And to your captors go the spoils.*

"Apartment is sold," I tried one more time, but again Hong insisted I tell the guardian not to sell. This had been her way with me for months, and it had worked, for whatever that got her. I hadn't called her brother. I had helped convince Dr. Winkler to take her off the pills. I'd had no certainty about what was best for her then, and I didn't now either, but worn down, I relented. "Okay," I said, "I'll tell them." Only this time I knew I could make no difference. She went back to her room, and in the weeks that followed, we became partners in denial, avoiding each other and the unpleasantness of our shared knowledge.

It was easy enough because I was busy. Patients were constantly coming and going, and newer ones than Hong were always presenting me with interesting symptoms. Like Mr. Bernard, the old drunk without a heart. He'd been looking better, but then one morning he told me he'd awoken to an ant attack, to the sight of them and the feel of little legs crawling on his skin. I only had a second to wonder whether there was an insect infestation on the fifth floor when he added, "Then the ant queen called."

"You spoke to her on the phone?" I asked.

"No, I speak to her through my head."

"Well, an ant attack sounds just awful," I said, curious about the visual and the tactile hallucinations, which I'd yet to encounter.

"If they come back, I'll jump right out the window to get away from them."

"Mr. Bernard, we're on the fifth floor. That's a bad idea!" I said to make a point, though the windows did not actually open, so there was little need for worry.

"It doesn't matter for me. I can fly," he said.

"No, you cannot," I said.

"No, I can't. I'm a human. We can't fly."

"Right," I said. But then he was off again.

"But I'm not human! I'm Greek! I don't have a heart!"

In the morning meeting I reported that he remained psychotic. "Describe this," instructed Dr. Begum. I told him about the ant queen and her subjects' attack. "Yes, formication—tactile hallucinations, they can be a symptom of alcohol withdrawal. So can visual hallucinations. Visual also more common with dementia, less common in schizophrenia," he said. "We were thinking Korsakoff's dementia specifically, yes? He will need long-term care." I started the Kingsboro paperwork. With all of the people we sent there, I imagined it like a clown car, with patients going in and in and in and it never filling up.

- - - - - - - - - -

Just as in the ER, on inpatient a steady cadre of admissions asserted they didn't need to be there. They were often believable. "That's diagnostic," Dr. Winkler reminded us. Everything was diagnostic. "Bipolar patients are usually in denial. They come in saying nothing's wrong. When they're not manic, they're very convincing." Bipolar patients, I'd observed, were also better related than schizophrenics, able to connect. Being with them felt different. Longtime veterans of inpatient wards had other, subtler methods of making the same discrimination. George had recently attended an intake on his own unit, after which a weathered psychiatrist interrupted a discussion about diagnosis to growl, "He's schizophrenic. I can smell it on him."

Differentiating between schizophrenia or mania—which were assumed to be organic diseases—and a psychotic character structure, which resulted more from early trauma than innate disposition, was another thing altogether, especially in the acutely ill states in which we tended to meet people. It would take an outpatient therapist some time to differentiate between the two, but who among our charges would ever have one of those? The medications were all the same anyhow. They worked in varying combinations and with unpredictable degrees of success on different patients. Someday the medicating might be less imprecise, but that was of no help now, to anyone I knew. Maybe to their children. But even then pills would be only a palliative, hardly a cure.

"I'm here because my stepfather called 911 for no reason," a twenty-year-old girl named Domenica protested to the treatment team. She wasn't lying. She believed it herself. Until a patient recognizes she has a problem, there can't be treatment—or so my supervisor had said, back when I'd had one. (Scott had found us a very nice new one, who admitted straightaway that she would not really have the time to see us and then made good on her promise.) While this made sense to me, it also implied a thankless task. If a patient's defensive structure—her very way of being, as natural to her as the breaths she drew—was built around denial and projection, how was she to begin to take in that she has problems and that they have anything to do with her? Treatment, it seemed to me, had to begin *before* a patient recognizes she has a problem, but then—the Catch-22—how can it?

Domenica could tell me little about what had led to her hospitalization, but her mother was more helpful. She reported that her daughter had a violent temper and that others in the home were afraid of her. Her moods swung, and she expressed no interest in doing anything with her life. Her mother was unwilling to take her back into her house, but she hadn't broken that to Domenica yet. "Maybe," the older woman kept saying. Domenica told me that she wasn't really her biological mom anyway.

"My mother is Beyoncé," she told me brazenly once we'd spoken a couple times, which made no sense because anyone who read *People*, as I did, knew the pop star was not ready for children, and she was just barely older than Domenica besides. "Gimme a dollar," Domenica demanded each time we sat down together. This is what babies would sound like if they could speak, I thought. Her visitors often brought food, which she shoved in her mouth ravenously and with both hands.

My favorite patient of the new year was aging and opaque, with a wide smile and a charming patter. He came in dressed like a businessman or a child playing dress-up to look like a businessman. He was too confused to give us a coherent picture of even his recent past—in psychiatric lingo, a "poor historian." He instructed me to call him Buck.

As reported by the case manager at his state-sponsored apartment program for the mentally ill, Buck's arrival on G-51 was preordained: fed up with the side effects of his antipsychotic medication—specifically its interference with his erectile functioning—he'd stopped taking it. Then he stopped eating and sleeping at his apartment, spending his nights and early mornings riding the subway instead. His case manager noticed his dramatic weight loss and general griminess and got him to the hospital. Unless he agreed to restart his meds, the program felt it wasn't safe for him to come back, and so far he was refusing. I was worried that he was consigning himself to a future at Kingsboro. He did not have an apparent care in the world.

Buck took to waiting for me by the door each morning, in Gabriel's old seat. "Hey, Doc, I need you to write something down," he would say. For a couple weeks I obliged, taking pages of notes as we sat across from each other at a dining table, recording the phone numbers of his bank, complaints he wanted to lodge against the city, stories of his time as a "certified peer counselor." I followed his orders to see where they took us and also because I felt for him. His hyper-cheerfulness and his social isolation made him seem so bereft there. He tried to make friends but with the wrong people—the young tough guys whose sheer numbers and strutting bravado often meant that they dominated the social life of the unit. They gave up only singeing scorn when Buck stuck out his fist to bump theirs.

"Hey, man," I'd hear him say as they passed him in the short, wide halls.

"Don't talk to me, you crazy old man," they'd hiss back. For these young men, I guessed, Buck was a cautionary tale, all the more terrifying because no one in the G Building would clearly communicate how they might actually avoid becoming him.

One morning Dr. Winkler asked how Buck was doing.

"He's less irritable than when he arrived but still pretty disorganized. His residence won't take him back until he's stable," I told him.

"He won't go back on the medications that worked for him in the past. None of the other drugs I've tried seem to be helping," he replied.

"I know," I said. "He doesn't like the sexual side effects of the Risperdal."

"Who can blame him?" asked Dr. Winkler. But I did not see how the all but complete lack of sexual opportunity inside the G Building beat out impotence on the outside. This was a clear case of six of one, half a dozen of another. For days I'd been thinking of how I might delicately point that out.

"We've developed a good relationship over the last couple weeks. Maybe I can convince him," I said.

"It's worth a try," said Dr. Winkler, "but we need to start thinking about other long-term care options, just in case."

I located Buck in the corner of the dayroom with his back to the other patients, his head down. "Zachary's at it again," he whispered to me. Zachary was one of the tough guys, in his early twenties. He dressed like a thug, but he was amiable enough. I'd tried asking him to leave Buck alone, but he denied hassling the older man at all, and I wasn't sure what to believe. Zachary was sitting quietly on the vinyl couch watching morning television.

"We need to have a serious talk," I said, and Buck followed me to the tables and chairs.

"I've got to call Mayor Bloomberg," he said, agitated, as we sat down.

"That can wait," I told him.

"No it can't. I'm on parole, and he likes me to check in," he said.

"Buck . . . ," I started.

"Where's your pen? I need you to write some things down."

I'd left my pen in the chart room, and I told him so.

"Well, go get it!"

"Not right now, Buck."

"Why not? I'll walk over there with you." He got up.

"Not right now, Buck," I repeated.

"Come on!" He waved his hand to set me in motion.

"Not right now," I said. He was thwarting my agenda, and my irritation with him poked sharply through my voice.

Buck froze. I'd satisfied his whims for weeks, never breaking from form, implicitly promising our solicitude would go on and on and never stop, though that could never really be. Buck looked over his shoulder at no one.

"Damn, Zachary, leave me alone!"

I looked to make sure, and Zachary was still twenty feet from us, impassively watching Regis and Kelly Ripa and their singsong routine. When I channel surfed past them at home, they sounded only half-grating, but heard amid the anguish of the institution, their merry voices taunted. "What was that?" I asked Buck.

"Zachary's picking on me again!" he said.

"He is?" I asked.

"You heard him!" said Buck.

"What did he say?"

"He said you're getting irritated with me."

Reflexively, I named the defenses in my head: introjection (taking a feared part of a caretaker in, as if to control it) and projection (expelling it onto another because it feels unacceptable in the self). No wonder I'd been so compliant. Buck could no more tolerate evidence of my ambivalence toward him than he could get the mayor on the phone. To know that I could become angry with him was too destabilizing. If it was Zachary who was claiming I was irritated, Buck could simply rail against him—an external enemy—and insist it wasn't true, which kept our relationship safe. What had he lived through that made such byzantine maneuvers necessary?

"It's not fair of me, but I *am* irritated with you, Buck," I said. "Maybe that's difficult for you to know."

Buck responded only with stillness, and I wasn't sure he'd heard me at all. Defenses are deeply ingrained, escaping our notice completely until the moment we're ready to give them up. Buck wasn't there—not even close. But if it wasn't a watershed moment for him, the interaction had an impact on me. Just like outside G, I saw, what transpires in the relationship between patient and therapist offers the best chance at growth. Not just stabilization, but a true getting better. Since my arrival on G-51, I'd wondered how to be a therapist to my inpatients, as if this were somehow only marginally related to being a therapist elsewhere. The ensuing self-aspersions kept me railing against imaginary external enemies of my own, a million little Zacharys. They drove me mad, but worse: in my need to pay them homage, I risked doing disservice to the people entrusted to my care. Holding on to my own convoluted belief that all that was bad and wrong and unworthy resided in me came at a cost, and it was no longer just to myself.

Buck sat back down. I told him I'd go get my pen.

- - - - - - - - -

The Justice Department was coming, and the paperwork had to be in order, and that could mean spending as much as triple the amount of time with my charts as with my patients. It was ludicrous, but like so much in the G Building there seemed no way of getting around it. One morning I went in early because it was quietest then and I had a stack of treatment plans that needed finishing. I unlocked the chart room expecting to find it abandoned, but instead it was filled with a group of skinny strangers, fifteen or twenty of them, and young. They were leafing through charts as if they were cheap paperbacks, and a schoolteacher, it seemed, was keeping close watch over them as if to make sure they didn't trip each other or destroy property. Someone with some authority must have approved whatever this was or they would not have been let inside, but the charts were filled with medical information that was not only legally private but, I thought, morally so. I was only an intern, and so it was not my place to say anything, which had become so frequent a conundrum that by now it made me want to yell. "What's going on?" I asked their authority figure.

"Nursing students," she said. They looked young for college, but maybe that was only because over the course of years I had suddenly become old.

There was no place for me at the table. When people began to arrive for the morning meeting, there was no place for them either, and the teacher finally asked her charges to stand up. They did but held on to the charts. Dr. Winkler entered and asked what was going on.

"Nursing students," I told him through pursed mouth, hoping he would become outraged and kick them right

out, but that was not his way, or he would not have lasted
so many years at that hospital, or maybe at any. He just sat
down, and we had our usual morning meeting but more
crowded.

The next day I walked onto the unit, and the same students were all over the dayroom talking to patients. There was
so much activity you couldn't hear the television, which was
lovely, and the patients seemed to be enjoying the flurry, the
closest thing they could expect to a party. I located Domenica,
the would-be daughter of Beyoncé, who was proving a difficult case. She was relentless in asserting that she didn't have
anything to talk about. Her distraught mother had become
equally resolute about not taking her home, as explosive
and potentially dangerous as the family deemed her. Until
Domenica and I got somewhere, or she was granted a bed at
Kingsboro, she would remain on G-51. I told her I wanted to
discuss how she felt about her mother's decision. It was painful to think about, and so she was ignoring me. This was how
it had generally gone between us. One of the students came
over. "Can I listen?" she asked.

"You'll have to ask her," I said, nodding toward Domenica, who shrugged at the student and grabbed the word-find
book the girl was holding. Domenica flipped through it.

"She's having a hard time accepting her situation," I said
to the student, but for Domenica's benefit. The student wanted
to know if she could ask some questions.

"You'll have to ask her," I repeated, my patience so easily thinned. Domenica shrugged again. The student looked
at Domenica as if she were an animal at a zoo rather than a
relatable human being, which on bad days was not so different
from how most of us who worked there looked at her, and my
anger intensified still.

"Were you ever abused?" the student asked, an especially abrasive way to begin. Domenica nodded.

"Were you ever physically abused?" she went on. Domenica nodded again.

"Were you ever sexually abused?" This time Domenica shook her head. I knew from previous discussions she was lying, and she looked a little nervous. I cut in, struggling mightily to be nice to this person whose poor judgment and lack of sensitivity I did not think lent themselves to her chosen field.

"Look, these are deeply personal questions. The answers are important if you're treating someone, but as long as you're just here to observe, you should stick with more neutral topics," I advised her from somewhere on high.

She looked at me blankly. "But they're on the list," she said.

"The list?" I asked.

"The list of questions we're supposed to ask," she said. I looked over at the schoolteacher, who was watching from a corner, and wondered what kind of sadist she was.

"Sometimes you have to use your own judgment despite what's on a list. If your nursing college isn't teaching you that, you're not getting your money's worth." I was full-blown nasty now.

"College? I'm not in college. I'm a tenth grader," she said.

I was lashing out at a fifteen-year-old. This is what the G Building had reduced me to: thera-pissed. It turned out the students were from one of the city's vocational high schools, which explained the naïveté of the girl I was speaking with, but certainly not why anyone had let her onto a locked psychiatric ward two days in a row. Patients could be unpredictable. Fights sometimes broke out. And what about privacy? This was no place for teenagers on a field trip.

"Gimme a dollar," I heard Domenica demand of the tenth grader as I walked away. I saw Buck sitting with a young man a few tables over and got within earshot.

"I used to drive a taxicab," Buck was telling him. "That's because I was a cer-ti-fied peer coun-se-lor. Write that down!" The openmouthed boy just looked back and forth between Buck and his list of questions and did not manage to get even one in edgewise.

As a substitute for comprehensive psychological treatment, patients were moved around, from unit to unit, whenever there was any trouble. Mr. Bernard, whom we believed to have dementia, was suddenly transferred from G-51 to another ward after a sexually preoccupied patient accused him of attempted rape when he crawled into his bed one night. Mr. Bernard had been getting into the wrong bed regularly with nothing more on his mind than going to sleep. He was just confused, and putting him on a different unit altogether could only disorient him more, and my book told me that such a decision should always be carefully considered by the treatment team, but that never seemed to happen. I was his therapist, for whatever that was worth, and was certainly not consulted. Transfers took place late into the night, or on the weekends, when there were no meetings, just the decisions of overworked staff who understandably didn't want any difficulty in their jurisdictions. Dr. Begum and Dr. Winkler were leery of transfers from other units for that reason. To be fair to everyone or maybe to no one, a kind of Yankee Swap developed, and challenging patients were traded back and forth between wards like baseball cards. Sometimes the reason for getting rid of someone was obvious (if counterproductive for the patient himself)—for instance, guys like Marvin Mavin, who scared people. Sometimes it was so illogical that you had to be there to believe it.

In late January, Zeke came from his rotation in the psych ER to our intern case conference eager to talk about a patient he'd just met there. The man's wife and two young sons had recently been killed in a car accident, and he had asked to be admitted in order to prevent his own death by suicide. Losing one's entire family at once was on everyone's short list of worst nightmares, and I could barely stand to hear about it. But Zeke was interested in hearing more. So even though he wasn't currently on the inpatient rotation, T. and Scott gave him special permission to continue to work with this grieving man after he left the psych ER and came to G-51. By the time the man was admitted up to the unit, though, shock or denial or both had set in, and he began doing his best to make trouble: selling contraband items like cigarettes, provoking other men into fistfights. Over just a few days he became very unpopular among the staff, who I assumed like me could barely stand to fathom the bottomless pit of his pain. Even though Dr. T. had followed ER protocol and confirmed the man's story with his remaining extended family, various members of the treatment team began to believe that there was no way anyone who had just buried his wife and kids could be acting like this, and they decided he must have made the whole thing up. It was likely the overwrought man wanted desperately to believe that himself, and the staff's response to him was a manifestation of this poignant desire. If there had been a functional psychologist on the unit, she might have called a team meeting to communicate as much and to defuse the situation; his behavior might even have gotten addressed therapeutically. Instead, a nursing aide came in one morning claiming to have seen the man on

America's Most Wanted the night before. The staff went on the warpath, trying, in a flurry of Internet searching, to confirm his newly alleged criminal past. Though they failed, the man had to be transferred to another floor, as our team's hostility toward him had finally reached an untenable pitch. Then Zeke fell on some black ice and tore his ACL and was out for three weeks, so the man lost his therapist, too.

I was often rushing between the inpatient unit and other commitments, and late one morning Dr. Begum stopped me as I was preparing to go upstairs for back-to-back meetings with Scott, who had begun supervising me on a new outpatient case, and Dr. Wolfe, who had proven the perfect foil to my women's depression group, encouraging me to enjoy myself and not take it all so seriously, which was good advice because it went against my nature.

"Go find the new female patient. Vera, she is called. We will be very fast, twenty-five minutes," Dr. Begum said. He was exacting and focused, and when I conducted interviews under his watch, they were usually brief, unlike with Dr. Winkler, with whom discussions meandered in ways that were as likely to be splendid as tedium filled when there was other work to be gotten to. I found Vera in her room. She was white and past fifty, in a gray T-shirt with a stretched-out collar, exposing her worn chest to her breastbone. Her eyes and lips were lined sloppily, which stood out because we rarely saw patients in makeup. She took all the time in the world getting to the edge of her bed and then rose slowly. She picked up a green mesh laundry bag filled with clothes and put it on a chair. She opened it. She found a cardigan sweater. She took it out. I wanted to encourage her to hurry but held back because her behavior was diagnostic, and I tried to stay patient enough to observe. In slow motion she dragged the cardigan's sleeves over her wrists and then followed me. Physically unable to make my pace match hers, I was ten steps ahead all the way to the chart room. When Vera finally made it inside, I gave her a chair and introduced Dr. Begum and told her we wanted to know more about her so that we could help her. We hadn't been able to read the admission note from CPEP, which was par for the course, and did not know why she had come in. I told her she looked unusually sluggish and asked her if she knew why this might be.

"I got two shots last night," she said. So much for diagnostic. Her accent was Russian. Her eyelids and chin fell as she spoke. I looked toward Dr. Begum. I had to be upstairs in just five minutes. I hated being late.

"Maybe we should do this later?" I suggested.

"Try a few more questions," Dr. Begum said.

"How did you get here, Vera?" I asked. Her eyes were now closed, and she didn't answer. We waited, and then I repeated my question. She managed to mumble this time, something about EMS wanting to take her vitals.

"What was going on leading up to that?" I asked hopefully. *Tick tick tick tick tick.* Her neck craned sideways now. A sleeping patient is a poor historian. I looked to Dr. Begum again.

"Why are you so tired?" he asked.

"She got two shots last night." I repeated this information when she failed to answer.

"They're fast acting, shouldn't last more than four hours," the doctor replied, and I thought that this was the kind of knowledge I was missing for myself and that it challenged my usefulness here. "But okay, you must go, come back later, we will try again," he said to me.

When I returned some hours after noon, Vera was more awake. She apologized for earlier, as if she were a student who'd fallen asleep in class. She explained she'd just then gotten her methadone, the safer and legal alternative to the heroin she'd been addicted to off and on for large swaths of her life. Methadone can be sedating, but it had worn off a bit, and now she could talk. She sat back down with Dr. Begum and me in the chart room and offered us a handful of reasons for her admission as if it were a box of chocolates. We should choose whichever ones we liked best. Caramelly suicidal thoughts, cream-filled auditory hallucinations, candied paranoia. But really she mostly seemed desperate.

"Where were you living before you got here?" I asked her, trying to orient myself to her life in the midst of the red herrings she seemed to feel were required of her.

"With my husband," she said, and she started to cry. The tears felt more genuine than the symptoms she'd been reciting from some memorized list in her head. "We just got married last year, right after we met. I've been locked in his house for months. He would only let me leave when I needed more methadone, and even then not always. Otherwise I was a prisoner. He was emotionally abusive. He liked to beat me up, too, to hit me with his cane." Vera's tears kept coming after she stopped speaking. I passed her some Kleenex, which she took to wipe her nose and eyes. Her makeup did not run, and I saw it was tattooed there. The artist had been one more cruel friend; the shaky line that rimmed her mouth was a millimeter to the right of her actual lips all the way around. She looked like a toned-down version of the cinematic Joker, why so serious. I returned my focus to her story.

"He beat you with his cane?" This begged more explanation.

"He's eighty-six years old," she said, by the by. She'd tell us later that her father had been high up in the Russian Mafia. He had beaten her, too. This is what happens to the daughters of gangsters, I thought as I listened, Meadow Soprano aside. Dr. Begum diagnosed Vera with major depression and assigned me to her case.

In inpatient terms, Vera was a real catch: she wasn't psychotic; she was angry with her parents, and that I knew how to treat. Her relationship with her father became the focus of our talks, which I guessed correctly from the beginning would be many, as Vera had no home to be discharged to and she was happy to stay besides. She liked it on our unit. She made herself at home there. If there was something problematic about that, it also seemed very glass-half-full. There was this resilience in her—in many of our patients really, though sometimes, in the midst of all their challenges, I forgot to take notice of it. Vera held on to the very human notion that life could get better. It hadn't been beaten out of her. She appreciated the unit more than anyone I'd ever met, and I felt grateful to her, really, for by then I'd come to dread the ward as much as the other residents and the staff seemed to. With my new patient, I'd found work to look forward to, and I saw Vera for forty-five minutes, three times a week. For both of us, it was nice to have some coherent conversation.

Her recent history we glossed over: cancer, heroin addiction, connubial captivity. Her distant past was more on her mind; she saw that it colored her present. Vera's father had introduced her to cocaine when she was barely a teenager, and then he called her a junkie and kicked her out of his house soon after they immigrated, and before she turned eighteen. She'd been witness to horrific crimes, she told me, things she couldn't talk about. Her father and mother had retired to Nevada, and, almost in their eighties themselves, they remained indifferent to her ongoing pleas for money and help. She was still trying madly to get them to parent her. The refusal to give that up stopped her from mourning all she hadn't gotten way back when and then also kept her stuck there. Our most intense sessions followed phone calls to the couple, and I saw that so much stubborn wishing died hard.

Vera made friends quickly on the unit because she liked to talk and she was also a good listener, which not all psychiatric patients are. She became particularly close with Ms. Anders, the woman who believed the American Mafia was coming for her. "I don't think it's true," Vera whispered to me from behind her hand for good measure.

"It seems unlikely," I agreed.

Vera got calls on the pay phone from patients who'd moved on, and she'd give me updates, like when a Mr. Archer called from Rikers Island to let her know he'd been arrested just hours after his discharge for stabbing someone on a subway platform. I kept waiting for that news to come back to haunt the G Building, but then I never heard another word. Vera and I had some things in common, personality-wise. My masochistic defenses—superimposed like paper-doll dresses over the depressive ones—had loosened over time in therapy, but I'd gotten to know them well there, to the benefit of my work with people with similar dynamics. My other patients often interrupted our sessions, and I guessed that they were envious of all the attention she got. Most of them could not tolerate a full forty-five minutes of engagement, and even the ones who could often ended up refusing my invitations to talk, like Buck, who'd folded his arms and looked away when I approached, ever since I'd tried convincing him to go back on the Risperdal. "Tell me what's wrong with me," he'd insisted, and Dr. Begum had come over and listed his symptoms.

"You are disorganized, you are grandiose, you are delusional," he said because this was the way some psychiatrists talked to patients, as if psychosis were diabetes or a gastrointestinal bug or some other disorder that had nothing to do with the unbearable difficulty of acknowledging reality.

"I'm a certified peer counselor!" Buck protested.

Like the most vehement masochists, Vera evoked sadism in everyone around her. She'd escaped an abusive relationship only to find herself in the middle of several fights in quick succession on the unit: the first left her with stitches above her eyebrow and the third with back pain for which a Saturday doctor prescribed Percocet. ("Is that a good idea for a drug addict?" Dr. Winkler asked when he returned on a Monday. That week's medical students said that they did not think so.) Despite my understanding of Vera's dynamics, in flashes of intense feeling I sometimes also wanted to wound her. One day she complained to me that she might have a roommate in the apartment program she was on the waiting list for, and I found myself asking, as though making a joke, if she'd been expecting her very own suite at the Waldorf. It came out meanly, as of course that's how I'd felt it. I might as well have slapped her across the face. While I watched her react, her placid expression shifting into one of wounded anger, Dr. Begum summoned me from across the room. I excused myself with a thin satisfaction and a thicker slab of guilt, like a repentant alcoholic just off a swig. This was the hardest work with inpatients, the corralling of one's baser urges. It reminded me of a physical fitness test from grade school—hanging, as they timed you, with your chin above a bar. In those instants, stopping myself felt like that, but sometimes I gave up and fell. These were not my proudest moments. Vera and I would go back to my comment another day ("rupture and repair," psychologists called it), but in that instant I was glad to be needed elsewhere.

In mid-February the Justice Department finally arrived. I would not have known but for the abrupt changes on the unit that were aesthetically reminiscent of a kindergarten. Multiple white poster boards adorned with many shapes and colors alerted patients to the myriad scheduled activities available to them. Trips to the seventh-floor gym, community meetings, recreation *and* therapy groups. Before there'd been only television, which no one had bothered to put on a Technicolor calendar. The group room was suddenly open around the clock with art supplies on its tables and one inmate or another playing its piano. I felt as if we were the von Trapp family putting on the final performance for the Nazis. Even the patients got in on the act, stopping just short of curtsying and exhibiting other best behaviors as the feds toured the building escorted by administrators.

"At least you guys will finally have some exposure to how a functional unit looks," said our nominal supervisor, who'd eked out some time to meet with Bruce, Tamar, and me as a group, now that the preparations for the DOJ visit had culminated. She apologized too, said she felt bad for us that our inpatient experience had been in the G Building in this time of a real mess. She herself had interned on a different coast, in a functional place. She'd gotten a lot out of it, she said. Our time on G-51 was winding down by then, and I thought that maybe I'd learned just as much or even more from seeing what happened when things didn't go well, when psychology as a discipline was practically as marginalized as the lunatics themselves. It was starting to sink in, the reality of it, that I might matter after all in this place, if others would let me—no, if I would let myself.

There was a morning meeting, and it was the usual. A patient was acting out, but we did not discuss it as if it were a treatment matter to be understood and articulated and shared with him to some therapeutic end. "I can't take him anymore. We're letting him go," a nurse declared, enraged, as if this were sound punishment. I'd heard threats like this before— not so different from my outburst with Vera, none of us were immune to these—though usually the line went, "If he doesn't stop being so intrusive, we're not letting him leave!" At home later I asked George if he thought all this was normal. He declared, "No!" but then reflected and said that even at his private hospital, where patients and psychology trainees were both better attended to, respect for our discipline was hardly consistently maintained. A psychiatry resident had recently admonished him not to speak to his patients about their lives "because sometimes it upsets them."

On my own I thought about why I'd gotten nasty with Vera in that particular moment. Something about her entitlement annoyed me. It was a trait I disavowed in myself, perhaps, but I wished I had supervision to dig a little deeper into the scenario. After some thinking, I went back to her. I asked how what I'd said had felt, and she said she'd been hurt. She recalled a time on the streets when a transvestite had spit in her face, and I knew then that my passive vitriol had hit her like that shower of saliva. With the transvestite she'd gotten so angry she blacked out, which she told me she tended to do when enraged. That morning a nurse had offered her new clothing, but she felt she couldn't accept it. We talked about her need to see herself as someone who got nothing, and how that got in the way of ever having a different experience. I thought again how much we were alike, just me without the psychopath father, a not inconsequential difference in our respective developmental trajectories, despite the overlapping defenses.

My last week came, and I said good-bye to Dr. Begum and Dr. Winkler, whose kindness I felt especially grateful for because it had not really been their job to provide that. I thought they'd be at a loss without us, but they didn't seem too concerned. There weren't always psychology interns, and certainly things went along. Around the same time George said good-bye to his inpatients over games of foosball and Ping-Pong, I had final sessions across sticky dayroom tables with Domenica and Hong and Buck—each of whom was finally Kingsboro-bound—and one with Vera, who cried and said she would miss seeing me. When I asked her what she'd valued about our time together, because really I wanted to know, she thought and then said that I had made her feel like a person again. The residents of G-51 had gotten so little from others historically that maybe it did not take much more than a little talking to help them regain a feel for their humanity. With Vera, I still regretted that I'd never figured out how to share my messy experience of being with her—that might have meant some growth for both of us. It was a hard thing to know how to do, and after all this time I got that it was the only thing that would make one that rare being: a therapeutic inpatient psychologist.

- - - - - - - - -

And then it was post-midyear, time for Caitlin Downs to share my midyear evaluation. She gritted her teeth as she greeted me. I could tell she was nervous as she shut the door to her office. I'd seen so little but bluster and nastiness from my supervisor it immediately made me tense as well. In a wavering voice she began with her anger about my disrespectful attitude, of which she gave examples—as if she'd been keeping a list and as if I'd argue the point. I had canceled supervisions; I'd addressed her as Caitlin rather than as Dr. Downs in front of a group of internship applicants; I didn't seem to carry out her instructions; I never appreciated the things she had to say. When she got to the last part, her voice broke. Her eyes teared. She said I'd been making her feel so bad that she'd been complaining about me each week in the junior supervisors' meeting (that such a thing existed was news to me) and also regularly to Scott. From their conversations, she'd come to the following conclusion: "You remind me of my father."

As Caitlin finally began to cry, I felt embarrassed for her, and I felt guilty. I'd seen myself as so powerless in the situation that it hardly occurred to me I was having any impact on her at all. I cringed at the personal information, which she seemed to want to be congratulated for revealing. It occurred to me, since we were sharing, that I might register my own complaints about the way supervision was going—if I'd been no fun, she'd been none either—but I felt so bad about upsetting her that I just vowed to be nicer to Caitlin going forward, to try to find something of value in our time together. Once during graduate school, I'd worked with a patient I really couldn't stand. "You have to find one thing to like in her," my supervisor at the time emphasized. All I could come up with was that she had pretty hair. "So focus on that," he told me. "Eventually, something else will come along." But it never did, and the woman finally left. She was the only patient I lost during grad school. Caitlin was not the psychologist I needed her to be, but she did show up for every single meeting. It was the one thing I could give her credit for. That would be my point of focus.

The next week when I arrived for supervision with my new attitude, Caitlin announced she had a surprise for me. She'd gotten me a new patient. "You can finally get rid of Carmen," she said, smiling. Carmen had continued to miss sessions, and I'd been frustrated by her absences for some time. Still, over six or seven months we'd established a relationship, and I knew she counted on me, even if she wasn't always able, for complicated psychological reasons we'd been trying to flesh out, to bear coming in. Caitlin was acting like this was a gift, but for me it felt like the opposite: an un-gift without a receipt. I tried to match Caitlin's enthusiasm to throw her off the scent of my horrified dismay.

"That's great news about an additional patient. Thank you. But I'd actually like to keep seeing Carmen as well. Cutting her off doesn't feel right to me," I said. I left out what I knew very well she already knew very well: this goes against every fiber of my being.

"No," replied Caitlin flatly. "She goes."

It was spoken like a challenge. Would I continue to question her authority even after she'd finally told me, through tears and no small amount of returned dislike, that she did not welcome such affronts? I had used up any slack I had with Caitlin a long time ago through ire and self-indulgent quibbling. This was to be my payback, a straitjacket of my own making.

If I could not continue individually with Carmen, maybe

I could see her in group. Dr. Wolfe agreed that was a fine idea, but I knew it was also an impossible sell. Carmen came only once and looked down her nose at the women around her. She stayed the entire ninety minutes, and when it was over, she gave me a piece of stale birthday cake—leftovers—she'd brought in a napkin from home. I left her phone messages for some weeks after. Each went unreturned, and I never saw her again.

CHAPTER NINE

tion in A Building on the first Monday in March. After twenty straight weeks of mornings in G—oh, how had I endured?—I climbed the subway steps at Winthrop against the backdrop of the singing alarms and turned right instead of left at the A Building. I cut through the littered parking lot of the BP station and crossed at the light onto Clarkson Avenue as I dug through my bag for my hospital ID. Since CPEP, I'd worn the card clipped to my shirt because no one can try to choke you with an ID that's clipped to your shirt. Now two buildings away, in another force field, I hung it back on its metal ball chain, the kind they put dog tags on, and draped it over my head like a tree ornament.

Consultation liaison was one more thing I'd never heard of during school, far away from the broader applications of my field. Apparently, it was the interface between behavioral health and the other medical disciplines. When hospital doctors have concerns about their patients' mental health, they call for a psych consult, and the consultant sees the patient and makes recommendations. Most teaching hospitals have CL departments, and they're often composed of interdisciplinary teams of psychologists, psychiatrists, nurses, and social workers. Kings County's CL team worked alongside that of SUNY Downstate—Downstate was the private hospital across the street, where patients with insurance tended to go—and was composed solely of psychiatrists. Still, because CL was an arena psychologists routinely worked in elsewhere, we'd been invited to rotate through, to get a taste for what it was like. Tamar had done CL back when I was at the court clinic, and she assured me that the psychiatrists there were friendly to us and to our way of thinking.

As if being far away from the morass of G weren't alluring enough, Tamar's stories of medical patients with discrete and transient psychological problems had gotten me excited about the four months I would spend at CL, traversing the hospital campus with great urgency. "Call for a psych consult!" a medical professional would yell with alarm, and I would appear to attend to the problem, to diagnose, and then to leave, never to return. I had gotten into psychology because I relished the complications of long-term relationships, but what I needed now was a break. Tamar had spoken of foreign (to me) and therefore exciting (to me) conditions: specific phobias, delirium, psychosomatic illnesses. And equally compelling, at this point in my year, was the fact that I would not generally have even one iota of responsibility when it came to helping any of these people develop further understanding of themselves.

"Good morning," I greeted the slouching security guard as I entered the lobby, lifting my ID to demonstrate I belonged, and he nodded his head to show I could pass, as if anyone might be turned away. The A Building was more modern than

G, with an actual snack shop up front, as opposed to just a window. I weighed my desire for coffee against the possibility of being late to my first CL meeting and then made my way toward the elevator, which I summoned with a button. Already things were simpler. On the fifth floor to the left I found the CL office, a large and dingy space occupied primarily by a wide, old table and a mismatched collection of plastic chairs. A long windowsill overflowed with unwieldy potted plants, and a woman in her late fifties wearing too-large, plastic bifocals and peach lipstick was watering them from a proper plastic watering pot with a very long spout.

"Good morning," I said. She looked up. "I'm Darcy—the psychology intern starting here today."

"Welcome," she said. "I'm Dr. Cherkesov. Not too many psychology interns choose to rotate through here. We'll be happy to have you." Her accent was thickly Russian, and her attitude was exuberant. "Have a seat!"

As I chose a chair, the medical students began to wander in. I could tell from their short white coats and their attitude of deference. They were always bright faced and shiny with anticipation. The phone on a table in the corner rang, and one of them asked me if she should answer it. It was her group's first day, too. Dr. Singer—whom I'd met back in July, that long-ago time, when my intern cohort toured the different rotations—arrived and took a seat next to Dr. Cherkesov, who had finished with the plants. The two of them made an oddly concordant pair. He was very late middle-aged and too thin by half, with military-issue glasses, boils on his gaunt face and neck, and multiple wool sweaters under a frayed tweed jacket. She wore her graying black hair pulled back into a severe bun, with upside-down glasses and Soviet-era lipstick that complemented her polyester dress, Dr. Cherkesov from the bloc.

Seated side by side, they were a pair straight out of a graphic novel: the kindly, old-world, adoptive parents who are soon left behind as the boy they raised goes off to confront his past on his way to a singular future.

Dr. Cherkesov welcomed us all to CL. I could read her ID card now, hanging around her neck, and it attested to her dual degrees: M.D., Ph.D. (Medical doctors could do an extra research year after med school, which earned them a Ph.D. "Mud Phuds," I'd heard them called, though I'd never met one before.) She asked us to go around the table to introduce ourselves. After we did, she explained that we would gather every morning at 9:00 to review cases that had been seen the previous day or in the middle of the night by the psychiatry resident on call. She turned then to the resident, identifiable by her longer white coat and her fatigue. "How was the night, Dr. Malou?" she asked.

"Only one call," said the resident. She was African, with a lovely lilting voice. "Twenty-three-year-old Hispanic female with no significant medical or psychiatric history presented in the ER after a suicide attempt in which she ingested Clorox bleach. She was oriented in all spheres. She was adequately groomed, slim, appeared her chronological age. Her speech was fluent and articulate, normal rate and volume. Her mood was neutral, and her affect was appropriate to content. Her thought process was organized. She denied auditory and visual hallucinations. She reported that she regretted swallowing the bleach."

"So you admitted her to the G-ER after she was medically cleared?" asked Dr. Cherkesov.

"No," replied the young doctor. "It was her first attempt. She realized what she'd done was foolish, that she didn't want to die. She had family to go home to, and that was what she wanted, so I cleared her psychiatrically for discharge. She left this morning."

Dr. Cherkesov looked at the resident with exaggerated dismay. She began to lecture, and her listeners offered their rapt attention. "When someone presents after a suicide attempt in the medical ER, they call us in to determine whether the patient can go home once she is medically cleared, or whether she needs to go to the psychiatric emergency room in the G Building for further assessment.

"When we are making this decision, we must ask: How dangerous and irreversible was the attempt? How painful is her chosen method? People think that Tylenol overdose is a painless way to go—it is not, by the way, it's really a torturous death. But someone who drinks bleach? She knows she is going to suffer before she dies, and she is more than willing to do it."

The resident looked pained and offered, "She said she got angry at her mother and did it on impulse."

"Even worse!" said Dr. Cherkesov. "Who is to say what she will do next time there is an impulse? Until you and the patient get to the bottom of how this happened, it can happen again. If she is sent to the G-ER, she will be pushed to process her experience. Again and again people will ask her about the attempt, and she will be forced out of her denial, her assertion that this is no big deal. Discharging her only reinforces that what she did is almost irrelevant." She paused. "Dr. Malou, you took this too lightly. The crime did not fit its punishment."

Dr. Cherkesov returned to addressing the rest of us: "A study was done of patients presenting to the medical ER after a suicide attempt. Those who were sent from the medical ER to the G-ER after their attempt were less likely to attempt a second time."

Dr. Malou was fighting off tears. I felt for her and with delicious dread anticipated the day when *I* might be on the receiving end of such a grave teaching point, one that I was never likely to forget. Dr. Cherkesov seemed to take pity on the young doctor and smiled gently. Her tone, if not her message, lightened as her smile broadened, and I found her so acutely and charmingly Russian: "Anyway, you discharged her. I hope nothing will happen. I hope it won't affect your life in horrible ways!"

Dr. Malou got up and gathered her notes and her worry and her shame. Dr. Singer began to fill Dr. Cherkesov in on a case from the day before. The rest of us stopped rubbernecking and turned our attention toward him. He had seen a woman admitted for pregnancy complications. Her obstetrician was worried that the baby was at high risk for cerebral palsy if the mother delivered naturally, but the woman would not agree to a planned C-section. Dr. Singer was called in to determine whether she had decisional capacity: Was she in her right mind to make such a choice? He'd gone to see her and determined that she was confused, in and out of consciousness, and unable to understand the consequences of her decision—apparently, the CL equivalent of unfit to stand trial. I thought about the baby and asked, "What if she *had* been able to understand the consequences of her decision? She would have been allowed to put the baby at risk like that?" Dr. Singer said no, that if she'd been able to reason and understand and had still refused the operation, the hospital would have gone to court to ask a judge to declare her incompetent for the sake of the baby. CL was more serious business than I'd realized.

After the meeting I approached Dr. Singer. He was the head of the department and so—in the absence of any psychologist, the same old song—would oversee my tasks there. Tamar had loved working with him. Like Dr. Cherkesov, he welcomed me warmly. His ID card attested to his M.D. and Ph.D., too. He explained that I would spend some days at Downstate and others at Kings County. Each morning after the meeting I would report to whichever attending or resident was "on the pager" and go with him or her on consults in one hospital or the other. He explained that consults were requested by medical doctors, who were supposed to fill out paperwork where they detailed their rationale for the request: for example, "Patient is not eating and is having difficulty sleeping. He reports feeling sad. Please evaluate for a mood disorder." Often, though, the details were sketchy. A doctor might just write "not eating" or even nothing other than "psych consult." Sometimes you could reach the doctor to ask for more information, sometimes not, but the consult had to be done within twenty-four hours either way. Dr. Singer summoned a graying Indian man who'd arrived halfway into Dr. Cherkesov's lesson. "This is Dr. Kapoor. He's one of the attendings here. You'll be working with him today, at Downstate," he told me, introducing us. I read his ID card: another Mud Phud. Rarely did I have this opportunity to feel so undereducated.

Dr. Kapoor and I rode down in the elevator together and crossed the street. The sun was shining and the air was crisp with the coming spring. I felt my mood improving like the weather as we walked across the drive and away from Kings County Hospital altogether. He told me that both he and Dr. Singer had done their Ph.D.'s in research psychology, "so we have a lot of respect for psychologists."

"Some of my best friends are psychologists," I expected him to say next. How much psychiatric disdain was he trying to shore me up against?

Dr. Kapoor told me that his dissertation had examined how doctors talk to their patients about terminal diagnoses. He'd found that the doctors' own anxiety about mortality affected their behavior. He asked about my dissertation and my background, and I told him. When we reached the elevator bank, he told me I should go up to the seventh floor to see a call that had come in that morning. I was delighted to be given so much independence so fast. Maybe some of his best friends really were psychologists. He gave me the patient's name, Valerie, and her room number. She'd just had her appendix out, and the reason for the consult was "panic attack." I should see her, determine what had happened, and then go down to his office on the fifth floor to report my findings. Reflexively, I began to review in my head what I knew about panic—the unconscious emotional states that engender it—but then stopped myself. I had before me only this beautifully uncomplicated task. A panic attack had specific parameters. I would determine whether this Valerie had one, not theorize about its underpinnings or help her place it within the broader context of her life. No wonder psychiatrists often seemed so self-satisfied. Dr. Kapoor said good-bye and headed for the staircase: he always climbed up, he told me, for the exercise.

I rode the elevator until the doors opened onto Downstate's seventh floor. The floors were shiny and bright, the walls a pale shade of yellow. Doctors in white coats walked back and forth purposefully. Nurses in pastel scrubs worked behind the desk. I wished I had a uniform, some easily identifiable evidence of my role there. Everyone else who worked at the hospital seemed to have that much, from the security guards to the janitors. I felt so unfortified, wandering around in my street clothes. I found my patient's room and went in. Valerie was maybe forty, light skinned and overweight. She was lying in bed, looking as if she was recovering from something. I introduced myself as a psychologist in training and told her I was with consultation-liaison psychiatry, that her doctors had called us to come see her. "I'm not crazy," she said. My appearance by her bedside was obviously an insult.

"Psychologists aren't just for crazy people," I said. It was by now a well-worn line, delivered each Friday morning by Alisa and me, with utmost discomfort (it rendered such disrespect to the cuckoos) to our fluctuating group of cancer patients. "Your doctor was worried you'd had a panic attack," I told the woman.

"A panic attack?" She looked confused.

"Did your heart start racing at some point? Maybe you thought you were going to die? Did your palms get sweaty?"

"No," she said. Did I have the wrong person? Had Dr. Kapoor been confused?

"Do you think your doctor would have any reason to think you'd experienced something like that?"

She reflected. She was an easy talker once she got going. "I did get upset before my operation. I was in so much pain. I'd had it for weeks and figured it was gas. I waited for it to go away on its own. By the time I got here, it had been a month of hurting. So I'm laying there waiting to go into surgery, and they'd been promising me for hours that I'd get some medication. But it never happened. It hurt so badly, and I started to get worked up. I yelled at them. My blood pressure went up. Since I arrived, they'd been constantly prodding and poking me and hooking me up to IVs without any explanation or pain medication. It made me upset and a little nervous."

"Do you get nervous often?" I wanted to be thorough.

"Once in a while," she said.

"Tell me about the most recent time besides here."

"About a year ago my son didn't come home one night. He's sixteen. I was worried."

"When you worry, or even when nothing in particular is worrying you, do you ever have symptoms like the ones I asked you about—racing heart, sweaty palms, numbness in your hands maybe, or chest pains?"

"No," she said. "That night I just felt scared about what had happened to my son. I went downstairs to a neighbor, and she helped calm me down. He came back in the morning. Teenagers."

I did a mental status exam and asked about her history. She told me she'd been in the middle of a shoot-out once, twenty years earlier, at a party. "Someone pulled out a gun and started firing. I live in a rough neighborhood. Parties can get dangerous." She hadn't attended one since, but she assured me she still had an active social life. I told her it didn't sound to me as if she'd had a panic attack, just a reaction to pain and the unfortunate difficulties of being in the hospital. That seemed reasonable, but was I missing something? Her surgeon, after all, had been concerned enough to call for the consult.

I reported back to Dr. Kapoor and asked him what he thought had happened. He guessed that the patient's anger had upset the doctor, who'd responded by calling for psych. "The staff use CL in a lot of different ways. They don't want to consider that poor treatment or just plain lack of information might be having an impact on a patient. They think that if she's upset, she must have a diagnosable psychiatric problem. I'll check in on Valerie later myself."

The next day Dr. Kapoor told me that he agreed: Valerie

had not had a panic attack. But as we sat in his office, another call about her came in. When he hung up, I looked at him questioningly.

"They want us to see her again," he said.

"Anxiety?" I asked.

"Yes, but not hers," he said matter-of-factly. "She's crying. Doctors often call us when their patients cry."

Dr. Kapoor let me absorb this and then continued, "And, of course, she has a psych history." Another phrase I had come to know well, with its undertones of derisiveness.

"No," I said, shaking my head. "I asked her about that specifically yesterday. She's never talked to a therapist. She's never so much as taken a sleeping pill."

Dr. Kapoor's face remained straight. I admired his unfailing placidity. He continued in an arch tone, with a smile on his face. "You saw her for fifteen minutes yesterday. Now she has a psych history." He was still amused, though no longer befuddled, his expression said, by all of these doctors who were not psychiatrists. It was then that I first considered the gulf between psychiatry and the rest of medicine and realized that it might very well be as wide as the one between psychiatry and my own field.

One night a woman showed up in the ER saying she'd ingested antifreeze. She was high on cocaine and alcohol. The next morning at the meeting Dr. Singer speculated that maybe it hadn't been a suicide attempt. Maybe she was just looking for a better buzz. He seemed excited by the novelty of this idea, and so I felt excited by it, too. "Do people use antifreeze to get high?" he asked. I guessed that he liked having students around: they would know what drugs the kids were into these days. But nobody would cop to knowing about the recreational pleasures of antifreeze. He made a note to call Poison Control to ask.

Dr. Cherkesov, whose intriguing tidbits, I was noticing, were often delivered like grand proclamations, said, "The combination of cocaine and alcohol is especially toxic! Impulse control becomes poor! As the coke wears off and alcohol stays in the system, painful emotional states become overwhelming! It's a lethal combination!"

The resident Dr. Malou reported that there had been several calls from obstetrics the day before. "They rely on us too much," she complained. Psychiatry residents did three months on CL. Dr. Malou was near the end of her tenure there and it showed. Dr. Singer explained that a young woman had come in a couple of years earlier on the verge of delivering an infant. She hadn't even known she was pregnant and insisted on leaving the hospital in order to go to her own doctor. CL wasn't called. The woman left the hospital, delivering and then killing her baby.

"Ever since, they overuse consult," he said apologetically.

Dr. Malou was on the pager, and so she and I left the meeting together. On CL, I was well below the psychiatry residents in the hierarchy. This was correct, I knew, because there was so much going on that was medical, completely unknown to me. But I resented it, too, pervasive as the psychiatry residents' attitude of superiority to us psychologists was no matter the setting. Dr. Malou told me I could call her Amari, and my outlook on our relationship improved. She was my own age, with a brusque manner but a pretty smile, and being on a first-name basis felt much more natural to me, though the physicians rarely used first names even among themselves. Months of "Doctor" this and "Doctor" that had finally had the intended effect on me, and any other title had come to sound pedestrian, to the extent that I'd felt an immediate and startling disdain during the recent presidential primary debate when the candidates were addressed simply as Mrs. Clinton and Mr. Obama.

Amari and I made our way across the street. First on our list was an eighteen-year-old diabetic girl. She was in the hospital after letting her blood sugar get out of control, and not for the first time. Amari read the consult paperwork as we walked. She turned to me. "She has stomach pain. Her doctors want us to assess her because they think it's psychosomatic, but that doesn't make any sense. If she's not controlling her insulin, of course she has a stomachache." She shook her head and continued. "When they can't figure out a cause for a symptom, they decide it's psychosomatic, and then they call us." She rolled her eyes again. CL was trying her patience.

"So if we suspect going in that the rationale for the consult is flawed, what do we do?" I asked.

"We have to go see her, and we can think about the case in other ways. Diabetes is easy enough to control for the average eighteen-year-old who's been dealing with it for as long as she has. So why isn't she taking her medicine? That will be our focus."

The diabetic girl was effervescent, happy to have visitors. Amari introduced us and got down to business.

"Why aren't you taking your insulin?" she asked.

It seemed like an obvious question, but apparently not one that her doctors had previously thought to ask. Hesitantly, the girl told us that she was Pentecostal and that the preacher at her congregation said in no uncertain terms that medicine was a no go. "I believe in healing," said the girl. Amari took a deep breath.

"Are you familiar with the New Testament?" she asked. The girl nodded. Amari continued. "So you know that Jesus healed the blind with his touch. But it wasn't the only way he did it. You've read that he mixed his saliva with sand and helped the blind man see that way? Jesus used medicine."

"Huh," said the girl. "That gives me something to think about." She sounded as if she meant it.

"Nice story," I said to Amari once we were in the hallway.

"What religion are you?" she inquired. It was a question rarely asked in my parts of the city, where a weak agnosticism was the polite thing to presume—if sometimes incorrectly. In East Flatbush, God was paramount, one more thing distancing me from the worlds inhabited by many of my patients. With a shrug I told her I was Jewish, because that is what I was, Jewish-with-a-shrug.

She said, "I'm a Christian, and I believe in healing. I've had experiences with it. But these religious men who tell their congregants not to take their pills are criminal. When they're sick, they rush right to the hospital and take whatever their doctors prescribe, but it's not what they preach."

Amari and I climbed a flight of stairs and emerged onto another high-gloss floor with pale yellow on the walls to see our second patient of the morning, a woman with MS. The brief reasoning scrawled on the consult paperwork was "crying." When we got to the woman's bedside, she explained that she'd gone temporarily blind on the subway, spending an hour just sitting in her seat, nervously waiting for her vision to return. Upsetting as this sounded to me, what had really done the woman in was that her husband—who despite their fifteen years together knew little about MS—did not believe her and was certain that her lost hour had been spent in the throes of passion with another man. This made more sense once she told us that she had five kids, the youngest of whom had a father who was not her spouse. Still, by the time we got there, her neurologist had already spoken to the wary man and assured him that his wife had indeed been struck temporarily sightless. Things seemed to be looking up.

"So how are you doing now?" I asked her. Amari had instructed that I should lead the consult.

"Wonderful," she said. "My sister is planning a family reunion. My siblings stopped speaking when my mom died a few years ago, so it's very exciting."

It seemed an odd thing to say given the circumstances, but was it psychiatrically odd? Was she being tangential or just cooperative? I thought: Doesn't she know why we're here? But then I realized that I didn't quite know why we were there. "Crying." We established that she was employed, that she had deep attachments to her friends and family, and that she experienced only passing difficulty with her multiple sclerosis. Other than the tears, which were momentary and understandable, there seemed no reason to suspect she was any category of depressed, which was probably the diagnostic category most closely related in her doctor's mind to "crying." We wished her good luck and went to make a note about the consult in her chart.

As Amari was writing, the pager buzzed. She picked up a phone and called the CL office. Dr. Jonas, one of the attending psychiatrists I'd seen at the morning meetings, wanted us to meet her on the cardiac care unit to watch her assess for decisional capacity. Amari hung up and delivered another explanation in her weary tone. "One more reason doctors call us: when patients don't want to take their advice. If someone doesn't take their advice, they're obviously crazy and in need of a psychiatric consult." She rolled her eyes again. If her eyes were her abs, she would've had a rocking six-pack.

We dashed down the stairs. I loved all this running from place to place. It made me feel so unquestionably useful. Side by side we descended to the cardiac care unit. The space was big and airy with glass-walled rooms and doors that slid open automatically. Dr. Jonas met us at the front. She was in her sixties and stylishly dressed. She spoke brusquely and only to Amari, as if I were not there at all. "Seventy-eight-year-old male insisting on discharge against medical advice. He had a heart attack a few days ago, and his doctors want to insert a stent. He doesn't want it."

"So how do we establish whether or not he has capacity?" I asked into the air. Maybe I was not supposed to look at someone so resolutely not looking at me?

Dr. Jonas nodded toward Amari, who explained: "Generally, the patient has to show us that he understands the procedure, why it's being recommended to him, and the potential risks and benefits. With this patient, since he's saying no to a procedure rather than consenting to one, we want to make sure he knows the consequences of leaving the hospital without having it done, and we want to document that he knows."

The two of them went together to the patient, and I followed along. From his bedside hung a bag swollen with urine, and it made my stomach turn. I had not gone into psychology to deal with bodily fluids. The man in the bed was a youthful seventy-eight. He was olive skinned and lively, with nails like a lady's. Dr. Jonas greeted him and asked if he remembered talking to her yesterday. "Of course," he replied, looking down his nose to show his disregard for the question. *I'm not crazy.*

His physician joined us by his bedside. She was young and Latina, with a bleached-blond streak in the front of her dark curly hair and two silver rings on each of her thumbs. Later Amari would tell me that she was in a band. While we listened in, the doctor explained the risks of the stent procedure: localized bleeding from the catheter, kidney problems due to the dye, a bad reaction to anesthesia. "But none of these are likely because they didn't happen with the last stent," she emphasized. Apparently, they had a history. She continued with the benefits: the blockage in his artery could be cleared, reducing his risk of having another heart attack, which, she said, was almost inevitable without the stent. Her voice faltered on the last part. His refusal obviously pained her.

The patient cut in: "I've already told you I won't do it! I've got something to take care of first, some business. I don't want to talk more about it, because it upsets me. I'll have the procedure in a month or two." He folded his arms over his chest with a dramatic harrumph. Dr. Jonas asked him to explain the possible benefits of the procedure and the possible consequences of its refusal. He iterated both clearly. "I know I could drop dead without it. If that happens, it happens. We've all got a number. If you think you don't, *you're* nuts!"

We left his bedside, and Dr. Jonas told the doctor that she was sorry but that her patient did seem to understand the consequences of signing out AMA—against medical advice.

"Well, I guess we're doing the right thing ethically," his doctor said, trying to soothe herself. She walked away defeated, and we went to look for the chart.

"What if he had consented to the procedure, would she have called us to evaluate his capacity if she'd thought he was making a good decision?" I asked Amari, thinking of her comment earlier, that doctors called CL only when they disagreed with patients.

Dr. Jonas took it upon herself to answer. "No, but the nurses would have. If they see doctors shoving consent forms at patients who can't understand them, they tell the doctors to call psych."

I headed back to the G Building at lunchtime reflecting on my morning. I found it all interesting and was having a good time, but it was hard to say what relevance any of it had to me, to what I knew or could offer or learn. Still, I'd been wanting a break from complication. If I was to be irrelevant somewhere, CL seemed as good a place as any.

Dr. Kapoor gave all his trainees a lot of room to maneuver, and soon he had me going around alone with the medical students. They were young and had memorized so much. I really couldn't figure how they'd done it. They did not know a thing about graduate school in clinical psychology, though, and because I was called an intern, just like the first-year residents, they figured I was above them, instead of just outside their hierarchy altogether. Newly released from classrooms and not comfortable being in charge, they decided to rely on me. This was a nice change of pace, and so I nodded as if I understood when they spoke about patients with words like "hemiparesis" and "sepsis." I went with the students Camille and Raymond to do a follow-up. All CL cases got follow-ups. The woman had a urinary tract infection and had become delirious as a result. Delirium was unfamiliar to me. It was a condition they saw a lot at CL, Dr. Kapoor explained, because it often appeared postoperatively and along with infections, especially in the elderly. "It's characterized by severe, rapid, and fluctuating changes in brain function. Attention waxes and wanes along with confusion. Delirious people sometimes have psychiatric symptoms like paranoia and hallucinations—usually visual, not auditory. We treat it with a short course of antipsychotic medication, and it usually resolves within a few days."

When we got to the woman's room, a sign outside her door warned us to protect ourselves against the germs inside because apparently she had more than just a urinary tract infection, and there was a cart holding paper hospital gowns. Camille handed me one. "People don't always wear these, but I'm a little paranoid," she said. Sign me up. I asked what we were at risk for catching.

"Nothing if you're healthy," Raymond said. "The danger is that you get spores on your clothes and pass them along to other patients you see who may be immune compromised."

Inside, our consult's roommate had a hacking cough, and I thought that we might get TB. One thing I'd taken for granted working in the G Building was that nobody was contagious. Our follow-up was surrounded by men in long white coats, attending physicians, and they paid us no mind. We would have to come back later to assess the state of this consult's cognition. We left the room and stripped off the green paper garb. As we did, Camille got a call from Amari, who instructed us to meet her on pediatrics. Pediatric ward: the very juxtaposition of the words made me want to avoid it. My friends sometimes asked how I could take hearing about people's problems all the time, but the kinds of problems I specialized in were largely self-generated and malleable. The rabbi marrying George and me was a chaplain on the pediatric oncology unit of another hospital. Those were problems I had less aptitude to bear. Upstairs on pediatrics, miniature people wandered around in colorful hospital gowns, and my heart ached predictably. Camille and I met Amari (whom she and Raymond called Dr. Malou) in the small office behind the nursing station.

Amari explained that the four of us would see an eighteen-year-old with "end-stage renal failure." I knew "renal" meant kidneys, guessed "end stage" meant grim. He'd had two unsuccessful transplants in the last five years, Amari told us, and was in the hospital being treated for an infection.

"What's the prognosis for end-stage renal failure?" I asked.

"People live an average of three to five years on dialysis," said Camille, "but that's just an average. It depends on how his health is otherwise."

"His doctors are worried he's depressed," said Amari.

We went to his room, but he was not there. "Dialysis," the nurse told us. She said we could come back in two hours or that we could go see him in the dialysis room. I didn't know what dialysis looked like, did not want to, but Amari was her usual exasperated self and said that she had no time to return in two hours. The four of us marched in a column to the appropriate room at the end of the hallway. Inside were two padded reclining chairs, each occupied. In the first was a girl covered completely by an afghan except for her pretty long hair. In the other was a boy, face exposed, plastic tubes thick with blood poking out from under his blanket. I tried to keep my eyes away from those tubes. He looked twelve and could not be our consult. I hoped that we would make a quick exit. Amari asked the boy his name, and it matched the one on her papers. Trying to hide her surprise—he really looked so young—she introduced us all and asked if we could talk to him for a few minutes.

"About what?" he wanted to know. Speech seemed effortful. He looked as if he was in some agony and that he knew it well.

"Your doctors are worried that you're depressed," Amari said.

"I'm not depressed," he said. He shifted in his chair, and his tubes moved along with him and he winced.

"It doesn't look like now is a good time. Can we come back later to talk?" she asked. She looked uncomfortable but in a different way from the patient.

"Not if it's about depression," he said.

We left in a flash, as if the room were underwater and we required air. I wasn't sure if Amari was supposed to try harder to establish some connection or get more information from this poor kid, or to what purpose any of it was. I asked her.

"His mother says he hasn't been taking his medication. Is he passively suicidal or just hopeless?" she proposed. I reflected on the meager difference between the two.

Camille went off to call the boy's mother for more information. Raymond and Amari and I found one of the boy's doctors and asked him for his impressions. "He's really dependent on his mom," the doctor said with some disdain, though it only made sense. While other kids were out navigating psychological separation, this one had been on an operating table getting a kidney transplant, or in a hospital room having his blood cleaned by machine. I felt angry toward the doctor then. If we were all angry and critical enough, maybe none of us would have to think about this boy and his horribly raw deal.

Back at the nursing station, Raymond and I sat down. Amari turned to me: "Present the case."

I had spent the last five months learning this model, but applying it to psychiatric patients exclusively. Of what relevance was it to this kid, and what was I even supposed to know based on our very brief interaction? "Uh, he's oriented in all spheres?" Was he? He knew his name, certainly, but Amari had not asked him the date or where we were. These questions would only have irked him more. *I'm not crazy.*

"Start with appearance," she said.

"He's adequately groomed?"

She shrugged. "Looks much younger than stated age," she said.

"Right," I agreed. "Speech: low volume, normal rate. Mood: depressed."

Raymond interrupted. "No. Mood is subjective. He said he's not depressed."

One-upped by the med student and his meticulous memorizations.

"Affect is appropriate to content," I continued. "Speech is goal directed, indicating an organized thought process."

Camille came back and interrupted our exercise. "His mother says he's been sad for two weeks," she said triumphantly.

Camille, too, was a conscientious learner. When one is differentiating among the depressive diagnoses—our immediate goal here after all—duration of illness was defining. A diagnosis of "major depressive disorder, single episode" (*DSM* code 296.2) required two weeks of sadness. Dr. Malou weighed in. "We can't rule out mood disorder due to a general medical condition," she said sagely. (*DSM* code 293.83.) "We can't really know."

But even if we could, what then? Amari spoke as if these distinctions were meaningful here, rather than just bureaucratic, and I began to feel the familiar agitation that psychiatrists engendered in me, with their unspoken insistence on the primacy of their truths. Who was this kid, and why did we all need to flee him so quickly? If that was happening with everyone in his life, his isolation must have been unbearable. We could conclude that this boy had an adjustment disorder with depressed mood (309.0) or dysthymic disorder (300.4) or depressive disorder not otherwise specified (311), and maybe based on the symptom checklists of the *DSM-IV-TR*, one or the other of these would be more technically correct. This was medical psychiatry at its worst, treating people like math problems, adding up symptoms and their duration and pretending it meant much.

We finished writing a chart note and tromped down the stairs to report to Dr. Kapoor. He said that maybe this was my first CL therapy case. He must've thought there was something I could offer this boy. I wondered what that was. The next day I returned to pediatrics alone to find that he had already been discharged.

The psychiatrists knew scintillating facts. Like: IQ predicts the idiosyncratic success of antipsychotic medication (the lower, the better Depakote and Haldol; the higher, the better Seroquel and Clozaril). Or: cocaine can cause a psychotic depression up to two years after the drug's last use. And: people in the midst of delirium tremens are at risk for stabbing themselves. ("Bipolars stab themselves in the stomach, schizophrenics in the genitals!" declared Dr. Cherkesov.) I was so impressed with what the doctors had learned that the things they did not think about tended to befuddle me. The very fact of my befuddlement, time and time again, stood out in my head. These people were authority figures, and yet I seemed to have picked up some things that they had not. Here it was again, this ridiculous fact. If it did not bolster my self-denigrating tendencies, at least it supported a multidisciplinary approach.

Two mornings a week Dr. Kapoor worked in Downstate's outpatient HIV clinic, seeing patients whose doctors thought they might have psych issues. His job was of course to diagnose them and then to prescribe medication based on the diagnosis or to refer them out for therapy. The HIV clinic had different policies from the rest of the hospital. Whereas the medical students and I generally traipsed around seeing inpatient consults as casually as if they were traveling museum exhibits, the clinic patients had to consent to our presence before we were allowed into the room. Most often, quite reasonably, they said no, and so I had already spent more than one morning just sitting in the clinic's comfortable waiting room with my laptop and my dissertation data while Dr. Kapoor worked alone.

That morning, though, Dr. Kapoor called me into his clinic office when I arrived. He was seated with a bulky white man in his early thirties with close-cropped brown hair. The man introduced himself as John. John was dressed in black jeans and a black T-shirt, with two prominent tattoos keeping company on his bicep, a colorful crucifix and a black-as-night shotgun. John had just arrived and didn't mind if I listened in. I took a seat in the small consulting room. John explained that his doctor had referred him to Dr. Kapoor because he'd been experiencing panic attacks. He'd been having them for about a year actually, ever since he'd gotten clean after fifteen years of heroin use. He'd tolerated the attacks for many months, but the more comfortable he got with his sobriety, the less willing he was to put up with whatever his body doled out, and so he'd finally mentioned them to his primary care physician. Could Dr. Kapoor prescribe him something to stop the attacks?

Panic attacks, by definition, have no discernible precursor. They come on suddenly and apparently apropos of nothing, and so it's easy for people who suffer panic to feel as if it's simply a random physiological event. I wasn't certain that psychiatry disagreed with this, though I knew that psychology did. The psychoanalytic take on "apropos of nothing" is that it is not "nothing" at all but rather some unacknowledged meaningful stressor that triggers rage. Intense anger is not something that many people, and panic sufferers in particular, are comfortable feeling, and the overwhelming need to keep it out of consciousness necessitates a physiological response: the shortness of breath, the sweaty palms, and the fear of death itself are potent distractions. Panic symptoms are a compromise, as unsatisfying as any. Their occurrence suggests specific unconscious conflicts that serve an important psychological purpose, and bringing these conflicts to awareness is the specific goal of psychological treatment. The panic attacks go away, and the patient has access to a necessary depth of human experience as well.

I wasn't sure what Dr. Kapoor's personal take on panic attacks was—if he thought they were meaningful beyond the physiological symptoms. Dr. Kapoor was obviously smart and also thoughtful and had tried to get me going on a "therapy case," but I had seen too many competent minds dismiss psychological underpinnings to maintain any faith that such an approach was always beneath him. While I began to think about John's problem in the context of what little information I had about him—his history of heroin addiction, the dueling symbols on his arm—Dr. Kapoor's questions for John did not imply that his symptoms warranted any further exploration. They were simply to be counted. Did he meet the criteria for panic disorder (300.21) or generalized anxiety disorder (300.2) or panic disorder with agoraphobia (300.22)? Whatever else Dr. Kapoor might have been thinking was not communicated to John, which would only reinforce the patient's sense that such a problem could only be treated with pills. The attacks themselves would likely become less incapacitating as long as he stayed on the meds, but the medication would do nothing else to help him live a fuller life. For the momentary comfort the pills offered, their limitations precluded so much that was worthwhile and less ephemeral. Dr. Kapoor would see John to follow up on the meds but at least for the time being did not recommend psychotherapy. I sat there on my hands.

I'd come to CL hoping for a certain effortlessness, a temporary engagement followed by a complete and permanent lack of involvement. I could already tell that there would be times when this would be enough, when all there was to say was "Patient did not have a panic attack" or "Despite tears, patient is not depressed." But I also already felt that familiar resentment, the insult to my self-esteem as I watched people who had more experience than I—whose very job I'd presumed it was to know more than a mere trainee—address something psychologically treatable as if it were not so. In this way, CL offered me anything but ease, at least for as long as I chose to maintain my lesser-than position. Student. The moniker had worn so thin, my last and sorriest excuse.

That afternoon I went to Scott to ask whether he might dig up a psychologist to provide some extra supervision during my time on CL. I craved my own discipline's perspective, which was the implicit promise of this internship and one that had been only minimally fulfilled. He acknowledged the soundness of the idea halfheartedly, and we both knew we'd never speak of it again. Later in the week I asked him for a letter of recommendation. It was March and time to think about what would come next, and there was a job I was applying for. Scott hedged in a similar way, and I knew it was one more thing he wouldn't give me. I left his office unsettled.

Dr. Winslow was the youngest CL attending, and the best looking. He might have been a catalog model for J.Crew or the Gap, and he was yet another CL brainiac besides. He'd been on CL at Bellevue before coming to Downstate, and he sang the praises of the interdisciplinary team there, but he never sent me alone on calls like Dr. Kapoor did, and Tamar said he never would. One morning I walked into the consult office toward the end of a conversation he was having with a resident. They were discussing a patient in obstetrics we'd be following up with that morning. "She has an outpatient therapist who she's been with for a while, but she's no good. She's a social worker," he said to the resident. His last sentence dripped contempt. He looked at me and smiled handsomely. He was really very handsome. "I don't know about you, but I don't think much of social workers as clinicians," he said with a conspiratorial glinting smile.

Well, the damnable truth be told, I didn't either. We all needed somebody to buttress our professional worth. Physicians had psychiatrists, who I'd come to learn were the scourge of the medical profession. Psychiatrists had psychologists. Whom did we have but social workers? One of my professors told this old joke, and George liked to repeat it: social workers want to be psychologists, and psychologists want to be psychiatrists, and psychiatrists want to be psychoanalysts, and psychoanalysts want to be tall. I suspected Dr. Winslow had no more regard for psychologists than he did for social workers.

"When you see the patient, tell her she should really be in therapy with a resident," Dr. Winslow continued, addressing the underling doctor again. Dr. Winslow was my own age and easier to challenge than the others, and I was starting to feel I'd earned the right to speak up, or that maybe I'd had it all along.

"If she has a good relationship with her social worker, maybe it's best if we don't interfere," I said. I wasn't sure he heard me.

The resident's name was Dr. Long. She and I left to see the patient we'd been discussing, a woman who had earlier that week given birth to a baby with Down syndrome. Dr. Long was gentle and sweet and completely unwilling to hear about the patient's feelings.

"My husband wasn't there when I delivered, and I felt so alone," the woman told us.

("Tell me more," I'd learned to say.)

"You're just tired," Dr. Long said.

"I'm afraid that I won't be able to take care of this baby," the woman tried again.

("Tell me more," I'd learned to say.)

"You're just tired right now. Everything will be fine," Dr. Long said, and the woman stopped her talking.

Yes, a resident, I thought, let us all have therapy with a resident.

There were often suicide attempters in the medical buildings. Dr. Cherkesov insisted on sending them to CPEP after and especially when there was a note. "If a person took the time to write, it's not impulsive. They're going to G, and I'm not changing my mind." Not all the CL psychiatrists shared her view. I went with Dr. Jonas—whose contemptuous attitude, I had learned, had made her the trainees' least favorite attending—and a resident named Alvin Wang to see a would-be suicide. She'd written a note. She'd taken some pills. She was sorry she'd done it. Dr. Jonas thought she was better and cleared her psychiatrically for discharge, and after the consult I asked the doctor, though she had still yet to officially acknowledge me, about her thinking.

"If they seem okay, I don't send them to G. I see what happens when people have psych histories," she said gravely. But what was it exactly that happened? They would feel embarrassed? For someone who'd elected to become a psychiatrist, Dr. Jonas certainly seemed to find emotional problems repellent.

Our next stop was obstetrics. We went to see a woman who'd miscarried at five months. "She's been quiet," her obstetrician told us. Dr. Wang would do the consult. We went to her bedside, and he asked her what had happened.

"My cervix couldn't hold the baby," she told us. "I didn't have health insurance, so I hadn't been to the doctor. They told me if I'd gone, they probably could have prevented this." She began to sob, and the three of us stayed quiet and let her. She went on. "Her face looked just like mine, but miniature."

"What are the disposal plans?" asked Dr. Jonas.

"The hospital will take care of it," said the woman, who was thirty and bird boned and still crying. "Burying her would make it too real."

Dr. Jonas nodded at Dr. Wang, and he took over. He listed the symptoms of this disease they called depression. Trouble sleeping. Changes in appetite. Loss of interest in activities typically found pleasurable. Thoughts of suicide. If she had any of these, she should contact her doctor. The woman told us she planned to get back into shape, to focus on work. She stopped crying. We left. When we got to the nursing station, Dr. Jonas was livid. She turned to Alvin: "First you have to tell her you have no reason to believe she will develop these symptoms! She has no psych history. You shouldn't scare her." But what was so frightening about the idea of feeling down after a profound loss? Whose apprehension were we talking about anyway?

Dr. Wang located the patient's chart and began to write in it while his supervisor continued to lambaste him. His notes were too long and so on. A snapshot of the delivered fetus— she had her mother's face, her bird bones, but in miniature— stared up at us from the page in the chart where it had been stapled, but we all ignored it and focused on the yelling instead.

Dr. Kapoor told me he had an interesting manic patient for us to see. After so many months at the hospital, I wasn't sure that such a thing still existed for me. The patient's name was Carol. She was forty and thought she was the Statue of Liberty; she was black, and she had HIV. We'd talked a lot about HIV at morning report. CL was often called for HIV patients, as the condition was sometimes accompanied by psychiatric symptoms, and there was also AIDS dementia, which came with global deficits that made it hard to diagnose, Dr. Cherkesov said. It was a complicated virus with seemingly boundless sequelae. Dr. Kapoor called Carol bipolar, though she'd been diagnosed with schizophrenia at seventeen. "I'm skeptical about diagnoses from that era," he told me. "Back then, blacks with psychotic symptoms were diagnosed with schizophrenia, whites with manic depression."

We arrived with the medical students at Carol's room to

find she'd just disappeared. This was especially curious because she was on one-to-one, which meant a nursing aide had been assigned to remain by her side, a cautionary measure taken with patients who were likely to hurt themselves or run away. Dr. Kapoor looked at the one-to-one aide questioningly, and she made a face like what was he asking her for. We all went back into the hallway, where the hospital police were already walking toward us flanking our patient. In moon boots, a hospital gown, and a light green foam crown—the kind they sell to tourists on Liberty Island—she was a self-defeating fugitive. She took off her boots but not her headpiece and climbed back into bed. Dr. Kapoor introduced our group and asked, "How long have you thought you were the Statue of Liberty?"

"Since October," she said. It was April.

"How did you learn this?" he asked.

"God informed me," she said.

She told us some other things. Her brother was president of the *Wall Street Journal*. She'd been born in France. We listened, and her sister showed up. I imagined the sister didn't want us around, gawking at her crazy statue sibling.

It was a Friday, and on Monday we went back to follow up. The Abilify had kicked in, and the crown had migrated from Carol's head to her bedside table. "As the delusion gets weaker, you see gradations of its disappearance," explained Dr. Kapoor.

I told George about the patient that night, half chuckling that Dr. Kapoor had called her interesting. "But she sounds it," George said. "A beacon of freedom. Give me your tired, your poor, your huddled masses yearning to breathe free." He was emphasizing the possibility of personal significance, of metaphor, in this patient's chosen delusion. I had stopped

at "bipolar." After so many months at the hospital I was dip-
ping into becoming what I disparaged. I was forgetting to
make meaning, and I needed to remember again. I went to Dr.
Singer and asked to be assigned some talking cases.

I had come to CL eager for simplicity, but having it was
not so comfortable. It was like a compulsion, this wanting to
know people and their meanings, but at least I'd turned it into
something upstanding, something I would earn a living at, in
a future growing ever less distant.

- - - - - - - - - -

After Scott rebutted my request for a letter of recommendation ("Ask Dr. Wolfe to write it," he'd suggested, adding, "He
really seems to like you," looking puzzled by the thought),
and after it became clear that I was not being granted an interview for a job that had opened up at forensics (Tamar had
also applied and been called, which stung hard), it occurred
to me that though we were more than nine months into our
twelve-month endeavor, Scott had yet to conduct my midyear
evaluation. I went to the other interns and learned that all of
them except for Zeke had sat for theirs many weeks back. It
was no secret that Scott liked Zeke even less than me, and our
coupling suggested no sunshine or cupcakes were headed my
way. I knocked on Scott's door to inform him of his oversight.
He said he had almost completed the review, which of course
involved paperwork, and that I should come back in twenty-
four hours, which I did, to the minute.

"You've been the topic of much conversation in the supervisors' meetings," Scott said breezily once I sat down in his
office. I guessed that must've been the junior supervisors'
meeting that Caitlin had mentioned back when she reviewed

me, the one she said she'd regularly complained about me in. I'd hoped then, in the moment's thought I'd given it, that she'd been exaggerating.

"Oh?" I could only reply, the air going out of me.

"Your work is fine, not much to say there, but we really don't like you as a person," Scott announced in his pissy manner, and then listed the general complaints that Caitlin had shuffled at me a few months back. (Hearing these, I felt almost betrayed because I'd thought she and I had roughly worked things out. Our relationship had remained unsatisfying, but I'd been trying quite hard to be nice, if sometimes through Cheshire cat smiles.)

"Scott," I said, searching my mind for who might've been at those meetings, "these grievances sound like they all come from Caitlin."

"At first they did," he admitted grudgingly. "Eventually, though, everybody else got on board as well." As if there had been a campaign.

But who was everybody else? There was no way Dr. Wolfe attended any junior meeting, or Dr. T. or Dr. Matthews, my weathered and ill-attendant supervisor on a family case that had anyway dropped off the map before Thanksgiving. Dr. Meyer from inpatient was long gone. That left my oncology supervisor, who'd not said much when we'd had our review, and Dr. Young, with whom I'd barely interacted all those months ago on forensics. I pressed Scott. He didn't want to name names.

"Dr. Blanchard?" I asked. (Oncology.)

"Yes," he said.

"But she never mentioned anything to me."

"When I questioned her, she admitted something was a little off."

"Dr. Young?" I asked, and he nodded again, not exactly looking me in the eye.

I couldn't help it, I started to cry. They were tears of fury, but not at Dr. Scott Brent. I was angry with myself. How could I have knowingly inflamed Caitlin that way? Why hadn't I been trying harder to hide my general feelings of cranky deprivation? Dr. Blanchard had noted them apparently, as I imagined had Dr. Young. I deserved what I was getting now. I'd set it up myself, like a table primped for tea.

Scott handed me his typed-up form. On paper his assessment was more measured, and just for a moment I took that in before this idea of being *disliked* took me over. I left his office tearstained and walked to J Building for our weekly intern support group. The review, though much overdue, had been perfectly timed. With the other interns and our group leader—a former Kings County intern herself—I cried as I blamed myself. I was the bad one. Scott was only doing his job. (Could I not hear the vicissitudes of my character style through those tears? That I would identify depressive defenses so readily in my patients only to miss them gone full bore in myself is a testament to how seamlessly they operate.) The others were sympathetic and tried to remind me that Scott was at least half a horse's ass. It had only been a few weeks back that the child-track interns, more incensed than usual by one or another of our Scott stories, had wanted to go to their own director of training, whom they adored, to complain about him on our behalf. We'd politely declined, touched by their concern for us. No good could come of publicly crossing him.

After group, still unconsoled ("not taking the milk," went the Kleinian metaphor), I called Dr. Aronoff, who called back soon. My usually staid analyst was apoplectic. "That is so inappropriate! How could you let him talk to you that way?!"

She rarely, and by rarely I mean all but never, spoke like that. The nice thing about someone who is professionally measured is that a break from form has all the power of a macroburst. Her words cut through my concentrated self-loathing. I had provoked Caitlin, but our dance had taken two to consummate. I'd been grouchy and unenthusiastic, but not without some reason. Maybe I could consider my own responsibility without absorbing all of it. For a change I could be outraged, but on my own behalf.

Dr. Aronoff's words lifted my bad feeling fleetingly. Warding it off felt like holding my chin above that bar. Still, the next night I got a high fever, and over the days that followed, I became sicker than maybe I'd ever been, ruminating with abandon whenever I woke up about my bad behavior and all those near strangers who reportedly disliked me as a person. Bad, bad, I was so bad. The stress of the year had finally toppled me, and also I'd been working in the medical hospital with a less than adequate appreciation for a frequent washing of hands. Two weeks before my wedding I was out sick an entire four days, my nose chafed beyond makeup's repair. It was almost better by our blue-sky marriage day, and as George and I danced and toasted with our families and friends, we forgot about our training for the first time in many months. The next morning we left for Palm Springs, and a ten-day honeymoon all but vanished the rest of the chap from my skin.

CHAPTER TEN

WE TOOK THE RED-EYE BACK FROM LAX, AND OUT OF VACA-
tion time I caught the airport shuttle straight to the subway,
hospital-bound. After morning report Dr. Singer sent me to
follow up with a Mrs. Guzman. She was in her sixties, admitted after a stroke. Her doctors thought she seemed depressed,
and my supervisor was honoring my request for a talking case.
Her speech was slowed, and she couldn't easily move her left
side, but she told me she was mostly worried about her twenty-
year-old son, who she said couldn't take seeing her like this. I
wondered if she was projecting. I encouraged her to talk about
her son's difficulty, and for a while she cried. Mostly I listened
and asked her to elaborate. When it was time for me to leave,
she asked if I could return the next day and I did. We talked
some more.

In some ways it was easy, this work with the medically, as
opposed to the mentally, ill. The bar was set so low. I only had
to be willing to hear about their experiences. Across the general hospital—and I'd been all around it now—support staff

and doctors were telling patients not to have their feelings. "Don't be sad." These words fell on the wards as regularly as April rain. It made my blood pressure spike each time I heard it in passing. "I can't tolerate your sadness," I wanted to teach them to say instead, because it was more to the point and would also quickly give its speaker pause. Sometimes there were just things to be unhappy about. The *DSM* had a category for patients who were blue because of new and troubling medical problems: adjustment disorder (*DSM* code 309.0). Dr. Kapoor told me he preferred "adjustment reaction," which is what the international disease manual, the *ICD-9*, called it. "Someone who has just had a stroke and goes around like nothing's happened, *that's* a disorder," said Dr. Kapoor. Yet being not sad was often presented to patients offhandedly as the only acceptable course.

Dr. Singer soon had two more talking cases lined up for me, each eighteen years old. One had sickle-cell anemia. The other had been paralyzed by a gunshot. I went to Dr. Cherkesov to ask for some pre-session supervision because I wondered if there was something more active than listening I should be doing with these medical patients and also because she'd fascinated me in our meetings. Every time she opened her mouth a gripping certitude came out. It might be a dubious fact: "Horror writers get their most interesting ideas from suffering delirium tremens!" It could be inspirational: "Turn all negative experiences in your life into learning experiences and you will stop being scared!" And sometimes she intimated an almost magical intellectual prowess: "I know things I don't know how I know them. I was born in U.S.S.R. I came here and someone asked me what is the tallest mountain in the U.S. and I knew it!"

She was a Russian Jew who'd gotten into medical school

in pre–glasnost Moscow against all odds. "They had quotas, only take 2 percent Jews in their class of five hundred. I got in by telling myself a tale that I would. The minute you make a decision, everything changes!" She told us that she and her husband spent weekends walking the streets of Brooklyn, six or seven hours at a stretch, to oxygenate their brains and fend off dementia. George and I spent our Saturdays the same way but in order to revel in the scenery—the Brooklyn Bridge, the incense plumes as they rose above the Atlantic Avenue storefronts. When I asked her for some general wisdom about working with sick people, Dr. Cherkesov declared, "If you don't believe your patient has anything to live for, they won't either!" which was the inverse of what I'd learned in graduate school and felt like a lot of pressure. She also gave me an article about demoralization, which it distinguished from depression in that the former cleared once its medical precursor did and was unlikely to respond to antidepressants (still, everybody was prescribed them).

I asked Dr. Cherkesov to explain sickle-cell anemia, which she said was an inherited disease of the red blood cells that caused pain and infection and organ and joint damage. She told me that the sickle-cell trait evolved in climates where malaria was common, and that while having two sickle-cell alleles meant trouble, being born with just one offered protection against that tropical disease. I went to see Alisha, herself with two alleles. The consult question was "eating disorder?" as her doctors could find no cause for her self-reported vomiting. But Dr. Singer said the real problem was that she was infuriating the staff with her angry outbursts and grandiosity. She'd refused to speak to Dr. Singer, but he hoped she might benefit from talk therapy and thought she might relent if speaking to a woman.

"I'm not crazy," Alisha said when I reached her bedside and identified myself. She was a pretty West Indian girl in a skimpy tank top. She was skinny after losing twenty pounds in the past year, about which she seemed neither pleased nor concerned. She wanted to be a model and showed me an album with old pictures of herself, posing. She was fuller-bodied in the photos and said she liked herself better fleshy, as per the preferences of her culture. She told me she vomited from her pain, caused by the necrosis in her hip. "My doctors won't do a hip replacement, because I don't have insurance," she said. Who knew if this was accurate—there was, after all, emergency Medicaid—but she believed it and was in a rage. She was an undocumented immigrant and near homeless, she and her mother having recently been evicted. They'd moved in with an uncle, who Alisha said was clearly unhappy with the arrangement. It was impossibly warm out again, and Alisha'd been left to sleep on his couch in the heat and her discomfort. Walking pained her, and she'd wet herself and her makeshift bed in the middle of the night when it hurt too much to get up, which made her uncle want them even less. Hospitalization had been a relief, though she would've preferred to be on pediatrics, where she'd spent long swaths of time since she was twelve. She was eighteen now, old enough that they could refuse to take her back. The nurses there felt she treated them poorly, though she swore to me that wasn't true. She stopped talking and gave me a deep pout. Could I be of any help?

I went back to Dr. Cherkesov with the same question as Alisha's (could I be of any help?). "She is your classic difficult patient," said Dr. Cherkesov. "You need to talk to her doctors and nurses to help them understand the angry feelings a patient like this brings about. In psychology and psychiatry, we know our hateful feelings toward patients are only human, and we can usually stop ourselves from acting on them. These other doctors are different: they think they're supposed to be above that, and so patients like Alisha leave them feeling ashamed, which only intensifies their hatred. Normalize it for them and they will be able to better help her medically."

"So just talk to them? Tell them to try to be patient with her?"

"And then go back to her and listen. She's enraged because she feels helpless. Encourage her to reframe her helplessness. She does not have problems—she has challenges! With challenges she also has choices."

"But does she?" I asked. She was basically a kid. She had a chronic disease. She was in the country illegally. She maybe had no health insurance. She didn't have a home.

"You have to emphasize the possibility of options. Someone with a shovel has two choices—dig or don't dig. If you don't have a shovel, you only have one choice."

The next day, at Dr. Cherkesov's instruction, I went to the morning meeting on Alisha's ward. "She doesn't seem to have an eating disorder," I said first, addressing the consult question. I explained my understanding of her to her young doctors, of her frightened desperation and her paralyzing helplessness. I explained that anger was a natural response that they could use empathetically. "Whatever frustration you're feeling, she's feeling it ten times over," I told them. They said they'd read about "the difficult patient" in medical school and took deep breaths and vowed to be kind despite her provocations. They thanked me for coming and requested that I see her again. "Maybe she'll be less difficult if she feels like someone who works here is really taking the time to listen," one of them remarked. I almost looked over my shoulder. Worked there? He thought I worked there?

I went to see the gunshot victim. Dr. Singer had told me his name, Nicholas, and that he had a history of bipolar disorder. He was only eighteen, so the diagnosis suggested he'd had some kind of pronounced early problems, but what they were was anybody's guess. It was so hard to trust the clinical thinking of the doctors who came before you, and when your own judgment was still forming, things sometimes felt hopelessly mysterious. Not that any psychiatric diagnosis mattered all that much for my purposes: I would see him only briefly to help him through a difficult time. In Nicholas's room I found him with his mother and brother, clustered together tightly. She looked too young to have a son his age, and they were striking, all of them, with dark skin and darker eyes. Nicholas rasped that his throat hurt too much to talk; they'd just removed the breathing tube the day before.

"So what happened?" I asked his mother.

"He was an innocent bystander," she said.

Bad neighborhoods, I thought, such minefields. Did his mother know—resent?—that I'd never had to walk them? I felt apologetic. Life was so unfair.

"His brother was with him," she added. I turned to the boy. He was younger than Nicholas probably, but just.

"We were at the playground playing basketball. There were some guys we didn't know, and one of them left, but he forgot this crazy ring he'd taken off to play. Nicholas picked it up and put it in his pocket—to give the guy later. The guy came back looking for it and thought Nicholas was trying to steal it. He took it, then left again. When he came back, he had a gun. He shot my brother in the chest and walked away." The brother spoke matter-of-factly. He must've told the story so many times by then, and probably it was a familiar one even before his brother became its protagonist.

"He seems more depressed today than yesterday," his mom said. The shooting had happened just over a week earlier. The doctors weren't certain he'd regain the use of his legs, but his mother assured me he would. I asked about his psych history.

"He's never been right," she told me. "He used to say weird things."

"Like what?"

"Like that he wanted to die."

"When?"

"When he was twelve or thirteen. And before that he used to see things, ghosts."

"When did that start?"

"When he was two or three."

"What was going on leading up to that?"

"His father was murdered in front of him."

It had happened down south. It was drug or gang related or both, the mother was vague. The family had gone into witness protection, where they'd stayed for more than a decade before moving to New York to be near family.

"He got into the wrong crowd," the mother said, as though he hadn't been born into it. She told me he'd been convicted of arson a few years ago and then diagnosed bipolar by a psychiatrist who'd helped with his charges. Nicholas was in and out of sleep as we talked. I asked the mother and brother how they were holding up, and they reported on the business of that week: getting updates from doctors, trying to convince the boys who'd been witnesses to testify before the grand jury. "They don't want to be snitches," the mother said. "I told them this isn't snitching. Snitching is working for the police. This is different."

The next time Nicholas opened his eyes I explained that I thought he might want someone to talk to after all he'd been through and that I would come back to see him again soon. He said okay but added that he was fine and didn't think he'd have much to say. Could this all be so inconsequential— a shooting, a paralysis—in the life of a kid who'd seen what he had? He spoke as if his circumstances were about what he expected for himself, which in itself seemed like something to talk about.

When I returned two days later, Nicholas was restless and alone. I'd been expecting to find his brood, to work with the family in the wake of his indifference. But away from the company of his mother and brother, Nicholas looked desperate, like a caged animal in his eyes. I didn't want to get too close, but he was paralyzed, so I moved next to the bed.

"I'm trapped," he declared, scratching mercilessly at his thighs through the white sheet.

"Can you feel that?" I asked, watching his hands. He shook his head. He had a furry boot on each foot. He asked for some water. I went into the hall, where there was a drinking fountain and small plastic cups. I filled two and brought them to him, and he grabbed them and guzzled. A Jamaican nurse came in looking full of all that might comfort a boy. She gave him a shot in the leg that he also couldn't feel, and he was irritable with her.

"Baby, don't get frustrated," she cooed. "Everything happens for a reason. Trust in God." She put a pillow behind his head, and he asked her to stretch his legs. "Your brother should do this for you," she said, standing at the foot of his bed, bend-ing his knees while holding his flaccid calves. The television had been turned—by whom?—to FitTV. A muscular Israeli jumped up and down on a step, exhorting morning viewers to follow along at home. From under Nicholas's bedclothes a tube poked out, yellow with urine. The nurse left, and I turned off the hateful set. Nicholas started right in talking.

"I had three nightmares," he told me, staring at me intently. "In the first one, I got out of a car with a friend. He gave me a gun, and then I got shot. In the second one, I got shot, too. But in the third, I was at my grandmother's house, and there was no gun. I fell backward and hit my head and was bleeding all over the place. Once I woke up, I was afraid to go back to sleep." He stopped talking and waited. I often felt dreams were presented by patients like challenges, material for me to sculpt something out of, buttery maple cookies or Disney figurines.

"What do you make of all that?" I asked. We are the authors of our own dreams, our associations to them as valuable as any therapist's.

He answered, "That I shouldn't be alive. I've done a lot of very bad things in my life. I don't want to tell you about them. Yet."

The "yet" chilled me. But how many very bad things could a boy of eighteen actually have done? And what happened to the kid who didn't particularly want to talk?

"I never let my guard down," he said.

"Makes sense," I said. He'd entered witness protection around the time he'd learned to talk.

"My family expects too much of me. They think I should be up and running around already. I'm going to let them down. People keep saying, 'Don't worry. It will be fine.' But I'm not okay. It's not fine."

With that he immediately fell to sleep. It was strange actually. I felt weighed down by his vulnerability and all that he'd
intimated so quickly, rapid-fire. I went to Dr. Singer.

"Eventually, you want to be future oriented with him,"
he instructed. "What are his plans, and how can he actualize
them? Acknowledge what he's struggling with, and help him
to envision a better future. I'll go see him, give him some
Seroquel to help with the nightmares."

The next day Dr. Singer reported to me on his meeting
with Nicholas. "He's still delirious," he told me. "What he
said to you yesterday may or may not be true. No point doing
therapy with someone in a delirium." He gave a little laugh,
not at me, but with me, and I joined him, only a little abashed.
I'd learned what addiction looked like, schizophrenia and
mania. Here was delirium now, feverish and abrupt.

When I returned to Nicholas's bedside, he greeted me in a
friendly way. His mother and brother were back. I asked if he
remembered our talk.

"Not really," he admitted sheepishly. "Well, maybe a couple things."

I could tell he was embarrassed, and so was I, and I didn't
press the issue. I listened as his mother and brother plotted
strategies to get the witnesses to talk. The brother would testify the next day. "Good luck," I told him before I left.

"I like her," I heard the mother say as I hit the hallway,
which made me feel guilty because what was I really doing
for her son?

At my request Dr. Singer and I started spending more time
together. Tamar had really raved about him, and doctors and
nurses from A Building to C obviously shared her regard. He

was the Bruce Springsteen of Kings County Hospital, and walking the long, dreary corridors with him was slow going and magnificent. Everyone wanted a minute with the man, to ask a question or to shake his hand, and I basked in his limelight, important by association. In whatever misguided ways the physicians tended to use psych, they obviously valued it, or at least him. It seemed he had helped everyone, at one recent point or another, with a difficult case. One morning we headed toward 7D North. Between exchanging metaphorical high fives with passing physicians, he briefed and then quizzed me.

"Eighty-one-year-old woman. Cancer all over her body. She was in the hospital for two months, very confused. She was discharged to a nursing home, but now she's back after just one week with pneumonia. She's not eating. What was the consult called for?"

I thought: not eating.

I said: "Depression."

"And what are we actually most concerned about?"

I thought: confusion.

I said: "Delirium."

Dr. Singer nodded. "Good," he said. "Now, how's your French?" Our patient was Haitian and spoke Creole, which I'd learned was similar to the Romance language I'd chosen to take up in high school. We entered the hospital room, and in my twelfth-grade French I introduced Dr. Singer and myself to the elderly woman there. Then I translated his English instructions for her. Lift your left hand. Lift your right. Show me one finger. Show me two. She did as I asked, so we moved on to questions. Are you at a museum? Are you at a school? When she answered both affirmatively, Dr. Singer said we really needed a Creole interpreter and went into the hallway to find one. (In all of the United States, perhaps only at Kings County Hospital could one find such a person simply by popping one's head into the corridor.) He was back in a flash with a janitor. Still, our patient had already fallen asleep. Dr. Singer roused her. The janitor introduced himself.

"Ask her if she's in a museum," Dr. Singer instructed.

The janitor looked at him dubiously. "She's not in a museum. Why would I ask her that?"

The two of them tried to reach a mutual understanding, but the janitor's English was not as good as his Creole, and explaining proved cumbersome. Never mind, Dr. Singer finally told him.

"I think she's been delirious for a couple months," Dr. Singer said to me. "Her son reported she's been in and out. We'll do an EEG to determine for certain."

"Why do the doctors order a consult for depression with a case like this?" I asked.

"They feel helpless, so they call us. If it's depression, we give her meds; she eats; they feel better. We're who they call before they call in the priests."

He went on: "Do you know this old psychiatry joke? A psychiatrist is called to see a patient. He gets there and the patient is dead. The psychiatrist goes to the physician and says, 'The patient is dead.' The doctor looks horrified and replies, 'What did you say to him?'"

- - - - - - - - -

If Alisha's doctors began treating her better, she seemed only to be working harder to come up with reasons to be livid with them. I couldn't blame her. The real things she had to be enraged about—an incurable disease, so many impossible systems—were for her purposes insurmountable. But the doctors, available and now inclined to help, them she could take on, fists at the ready. And also, there was me, another passerby she could lash out at. Reframe her problems as challenges, give her choices, Dr. Cherkesov had counseled. But so far I'd only managed to become one more in a series of nameless, faceless receptacles for her hate. She barely looked at me as she seethed, in forty-five-minute stretches.

"My doctors are lying to me. They say my bones are still growing and so they can't do the hip replacement," she said for the third time in as many visits. I asked what I thought was an innocuous factual question in response, trying to remain engaged, only to have her spit at me, "That's a dumb question. I've told you this story three times!"

"I'm glad you're bringing that up," I said, speaking slowly to give her rage time to work its way out of me. "I must admit I've been wondering why you tell me the same thing every time I come to see you, all these times in a row." If she moved past her paranoia, what awaited her was worse. I knew that and she knew that, but we had different ideas about what to do with that knowing, with her preferring to stay stuck like a needle in a scratched record, and my hoping to keep her company as she acclimated to reality and its tragic limitations. I hated that this was the best I could do for her—anything short of a cure and a winning lottery ticket felt insufficient—but at least one of us had to move past our infantile grandiosity, our certain hope that we could conjure all we needed from the magic of our minds.

"Right. Fine. Well, I'll never tell it to you again. Obviously, I should be keeping it to myself," she huffed.

"It's not that," I said. "I'm here to listen to whatever you need to tell me. But our time together is limited, and I was just thinking we could use it more productively."

"Well, I'm sorry I spoke to you at all. To any of you! I came to this country when I was twelve because my mom said I could get better medical help here, and look how I end up!"

"Uncured and insufficiently cared for," I said.

Alisha's anger broke like a felled horse, and she cried then. I sat quietly until she asked me to go. Too spent now to hiss, she said it almost gently.

In between talking cases I was still going around with the doctor on the pager. On the irritable Dr. Jonas's days this was trying, as she was in a perpetual rush and three months in she was still acting as if I didn't exist. One morning I arrived on the fifth floor early only to find her already dashing out with her resident, Alvin Wang. Alvin smiled and waved toward me as he tried to keep up with his mentor's driven march toward the stairwell. Though by then she must've known it was my assignment to follow her, she did not slow when she saw me. A psychology trainee wasn't worth acknowledging, let alone waiting for. I went into the meeting, and after it ended, I decided to stay in the cool of the Kings County room rather than track her down across the street, but then I felt as if I were playing hooky, and also there was the nagging disappointment of possibly missing out on one valuable lesson or another. I crossed over to Downstate and found her and Alvin leaving their sunny suite of CL offices. They were on their way somewhere, and I fell into step alongside.

"Seventeen-year-old Hispanic female," Alvin told me as we moved along the shiny corridors. Downstate was as sparkling as Kings County was dull. "Raised in the projects. History of multiple rapes. Her doctors can't find a reason for her headaches, and they want us to determine if they're psychosomatic."

"If the psychology intern had been here earlier, she would have known that," Dr. Jonas said to Alvin, not looking at me still. I was taken aback, mostly surprised that she'd noticed both my current presence and my earlier absence.

"Well, thanks for filling me in," I said to Alvin with forced cheer. He grinned at me behind his instructor's back.

The three of us arrived at the chart room off the nursing station on the pediatric ward. Dr. Jonas took the girl's chart and scanned it. "She's got meningitis," she said. "Explains the headaches." So much for the consult question. She kept reading, and when she spoke again, she sounded contemptuous. "She says that she's had eleven sexual partners in the last month. She's lying."

With a history of multiple rapes, eleven men in one month fit. It wasn't unusual for sexual assault victims to become promiscuous in the aftermath—a valiant attempt to mitigate the trauma, to better understand or control it this time around. This was hardly an esoteric principle. Was Dr. Jonas really so unfamiliar with it?

We entered the seventeen-year-old's room. Yanibel was cornrowed and cherubic, holding a denim-clad teddy bear. "What's its name?" Dr. Jonas asked Yanibel after introducing herself, pointing to the bear.

"Miranda," replied Yanibel, smiling and batting her eyelids.

"If she's a girl, why is she wearing blue and not pink?" asked Dr. Jonas with her usual conversational flair. Yanibel gave an equally meaningless answer.

"So your doctors are concerned about you. They asked me to come make sure you're doing okay," Dr. Jonas explained. Yanibel nodded.

"Have you had the condom lecture?" asked Dr. Jonas.

"Yes." The girl was solemn.

"Then I'm not going to give you that lecture. Do you use them?"

"Yes."

"All the time?"

"Yes," said the girl, all sweetness and long lashes.

"Yanibel, I want to explain something to you. Sometimes teenagers have very high sex drives," she said. "It can be hard to control. But we have medicines that can help, like the birth control pill."

The patient was as attentive as I was horrified. Given the neighborhood, ours might be the only conversation this girl would ever have with anyone in the mental health field. If she bought the idea that her sexual acting out was simply the result of hormones gone wild, like soused girls in low-budget Mardi Gras films, she might never get it, the import of dealing with her suffering. I couldn't let this one go. I might have been only a student—for how much longer was that anyway?—but still I had something to offer. I could condemn myself in my head or fail to stand up for myself in meetings with people like Caitlin and Scott, but I could not let my oldest vulnerabilities get in the way of my actual work. I was not always bad. I was not always wrong. To regress into believing otherwise was to shirk a real responsibility—one it was time to start embracing, as long as I was there.

I interrupted Dr. Jonas with the indignation of a thousand condescended-to psychologists. "Can I ask a question?"

She looked at me with exaggerated surprise. "What is it?"

I avoided her gaze—finally settled on me—and focused on Yanibel instead.

"Did you have a lot of sex before the rapes, Yanibel, or not until after?"

Yanibel giggled as she replied, "After." She turned back to Dr. Jonas and her imperious authority. "Why is she asking me that?"

Dr. Jonas swiveled to face Yanibel, carefully enunciating each syllable of her reply. "Why don't you ask the psychology intern? She's the one who wants to know."

Her hostility threw me, but less than the realization that she did not follow my line of thought. I'd mistaken her arrogance for knowledge. That was so easy for me to do. My heart racing with anger and something else more exciting, I addressed Yanibel. "It's common for girls who've been raped to become very promiscuous afterward. It's one way of trying to cope with all the frightening feelings that come from being assaulted," I said slowly, hoping she would get it.

"Oh," said Yanibel. She stopped her giggling.

"Sometimes people go talk to therapists to work out feelings like those," I told her.

Dr. Jonas cut in, still dismissive. "We can help you find someone to talk to, if that's what you want." Her pager began to beep.

"Yes, I'd like that," said Yanibel.

"I have to take this page. I'll make a note in the chart for your social worker to find you a therapist, and Dr. Wang will finish up here." She left, rushing again, as if someone might drop dead if the psychiatrist didn't get there quickly enough. Alvin took over.

"So there are several oral contraceptives I can prescribe that may dampen your urge to have sex," Alvin began.

"Dr. Wang," I said pointedly, looking him in the eye.

"Right," he said. "That's not really the issue here?"

"No," I said, shaking my head.

"We'll be helping to make you a therapy appointment," he corrected himself.

"Good luck, Yanibel," I said. "Feel better."

We left the room. Alvin asked me to recommend some basic psychology reading to him, and I told him I'd make a list. We went to wait for Dr. Jonas in the chart room.

"You're good with adolescents," Dr. Jonas said to me when she arrived. "Do you have a lot of experience with them?"

I did not, and I told her so. "I've had course work on trauma," I added, hoping to communicate that the rudimentary knowledge I'd imparted to this patient had nothing to do with studying teenagers, but rather with my general knowledge of psychological functioning.

"Well, I think that you should consider specializing in teens," she said, trying to be generous, I knew, but also missing my point. Dr. Jonas stopped ignoring me after that, and I stopped ignoring myself, too.

- - - - - - - - -

One day as we waited for morning report, a young, blond medical student I'd been traipsing around the hospital with told me he was thinking about going to see a therapist. "A psychoanalyst," he added. "Psychoanalysis sounds interesting."

Dr. Cherkesov chimed from the windowsill and her plants. "You should go for something else," she said. "Like DBT!" Dialectical behavior therapy was all the rage in psychotherapy research circles, but it was primarily for managing personality disorders, and this medical student was hardly that sick.

"Nah!" I said, because summer was coming and the mood

in the room felt playful. "He's in the neurotic range. Psycho-analysis seems right."

"'That's a horrible word, 'neurotic,'" Dr. Cherkesov responded with her typical fervor.

"I guess it used to be," I said. "But not anymore. Now it's good. Healthy. High functioning."

"Well, the public doesn't see it that way," she said.

"I don't talk to the public that way," I said, defensive. "Just other people in the field."

"Still, if you believe that a patient is neurotic, your negative attitude is communicated."

"But I don't think it's negative. It's practically cause for celebration!" It was easy to adopt her exuberant demeanor, and fun.

Dr. Cherkesov continued: "Your words matter. Someone is not 'obsessive.' He is 'conscientious'!"

"But I don't think 'obsessive' is negative either. Everyone has a character style. It's only problematic when it repeatedly gets in someone's way."

"You will communicate your negative feelings about the patient in your face, in your body language," said Dr. Cherkesov, who saw the world in shades of grave.

The medical student cut in and changed the subject. Later he told me he did it on purpose. "I couldn't take the tension anymore," he said.

In the meeting that followed, we discussed a man in the hospital after a car accident. He'd been driving and was largely physically unscathed, but his sister, in the passenger seat, had been killed. CL was called late in the night to tell him of her passing. The resident had gone to see him. "Bringing psychiatry in to deliver news makes people think they're expected to go crazy," said Dr. Cherkesov, shaking her head. We needed to arrive at a psychiatric diagnosis so that he could be followed up. Somebody took out the *DSM* to look up "bereavement," and I felt as if we were a group of aliens investigating the human experience.

I left the meeting and went to see Nicholas, who'd become a three-times-a-week patient. He was a likable kid, but his self-professed sociopathy kept me wary of each confidence. When I got to his room, he was in his bed as usual, but now there was a slim black wheelchair beside him, and it did things to my stomach, imagining him in it. His nightmares had continued, and he shared them with me on each visit, revision after revision of the afternoon of his shooting. In the most recent iteration, he'd been watching his friends play ball from the sidelines, desperate but unable to get into the game. Did he still belong among them? He told me he'd been a drug kingpin. Those were his words, though I presumed the title an inflated one, given his youth. I didn't know much about street crime, but I'd watched each season of *The Wire*, and the kids his age were middling players, if always with the bleak promise of ascension. Nicholas was convinced he was bad to the bone. "I'm evil and karma made me get shot, but karma messed up and I didn't die. I've always known I'd die by a shooting, but I never thought I'd wind up like this." He told me his goal in life had been to be feared, and that he'd achieved it, but now maybe he was rethinking things. No one feared a guy in a chair. His mom had started talking about moving again, to get Nicholas away from this latest bad crowd.

"But the place doesn't make the man," I told him. "Maybe it's time to start being curious about your attraction to dangerous people." I wanted to help him recognize that repeating the life of one's father was a choice. Maybe there were other choices. I asked him if he'd thought of any.

"This gym teacher came to visit my juvenile detention class once. He'd been in a gang, but he turned his life around. We all really liked him. Ever since then I've thought about becoming a gym teacher, influencing kids like that. It's been in the back of my mind," he said. Was that where this shooting might eventually land him, in a junior high school gymnasium, not dead at all? We both looked at the wheelchair. He spoke again: "I had another dream, too, about going around to visit a bunch of different people. I told them, 'I'm walking, but don't worry, it's just a dream.' "

- - - - - - - - -

After Memorial Day, Dr. Cherkesov went on vacation, and Dr. Singer was overwhelmed with calls. "We'll have to split up the consults between the residents and Dr. Jonas and me," he told us at the meeting's end, unusually harried. Unlike Dr. Kapoor's, Dr. Singer's style was to see each consult in advance of the resident, to make sure he had a general handle on it before passing it along.

"You can give me a few as well," I said with confidence.

Dr. Singer thought for a minute. "No, it might just have to be the resident," he said finally, apologetic.

I felt the smart of his decision, but only for a flash because then there was this: I had volunteered to go. I had spoken right up. But where is the schoolgirl that used to be me? All year long I'd tiptoed around, revering the idea that I was lacking in some vague way that made me less than useful. Finally I wanted to laugh out loud at that very notion, the wrong answer to the wrong question. My offer to help out, delivered without hesitation, seemed more important than any response it elicited.

I was still very new to much of this. I still had a lot to

learn. But that mattered less in the end than the fact that I'd become willing to participate. It made me a better psychologist.

I ran into Scott on the sixth floor, and he stopped me. "I have some news I think you'll like hearing," he said. "I heard through the grapevine that you're doing a great job on your family case." He paused and waited for my appreciation. I'd been refusing to give it to him for so long (so strongly did I resent being asked to pretend that it was there). How much smoother my year might have been had I relented sooner. I smiled.

"Wow, that's really nice to hear," I said. It might've been, too, had I actually been seeing a family.

"I thought you'd want to know," he said.

"Yes, thank you," I said. As I kept smiling, I tried to figure out what might have gone down. Was this my good-humored family supervisor's winking attempt to help me out with Scott? So separate was he from the G Building in his child and family clinic, would he have even known I needed the boost?

"How's the paperwork going?" Scott asked. With just weeks to go, whatever outpatient notes we hadn't been keeping up with during the year had to be attended to. In our free time the interns were now camped out in our office together, mildly nostalgic for each other and this mess of a place, hands cramping as we wrote vague near-paragraphs about sessions long since past.

"Good," I told Scott. "I'm almost done." I was.

Alisha would go home soon, or maybe there would be an operation. The former was problematic, as she was having trouble keeping her pain medication down, and without it she was writhing and miserable. As an outpatient, too, it was hard to afford the meds. She'd borrowed from a favorite teacher for them in the past, but they were two hundred dollars a month, and she couldn't keep asking. Again I felt the heft of reality, this medium I couldn't alter. Maybe Alisha could use a psychologist, but there was so much else she had to have first. The teacher came to visit and stopped me in the hallway.

"I feel bad for her, of course, but she's really difficult," the woman said in a low voice. "She lies. She's manipulative."

"Think of everything she needs and can't get," I said to her. "Manipulation is adaptive in her case. How else would a girl in her shoes get by?"

The teacher thanked me for the reminder and took a deep breath before entering the room.

The next time I saw Alisha she told me again about her pain and her doctors' obfuscations, and I was empathetic and reflected how hard her struggle was. She told me she was glad to have me to talk to. Two days later I returned and she was gone. This was how treatments ended at hospitals, without the thoughtful summations and labored in-office good-byes I'd been taught to call termination. In all of these settings that in school had escaped me, there were rarely neat farewells.

Nicholas was leaving, too, before me. He was in physical therapy each day by then, not walking yet but making progress and recovered from his surgery. He would be transferred to a long-term rehab facility in uptown Manhattan, his mother housed in an apartment nearby. They were still talking about moving back west, but my patient had become

ambivalent, for from his hospital bed with his useless legs he'd
managed to fall in love. She was a few years older, a friend of
a friend. For a girl longing for a drug kingpin with the loyalty
of a schoolboy, an outlaw with a newly acquired heart of gold,
I guessed Nicholas was a rare find. At least carousing would
be hard from an inpatient rehab, for the months he'd likely
be there. The girl had asked Nicholas to be exclusive, and
he'd eagerly agreed. "I don't want to talk about anything dark
today," he told me at the start of our last visit. His face was lit
with the elation of new love, more potent than the Seroquel.
I wished him well.

As on inpatient, there was no evaluation at CL. Psychiatrists
did not evaluate psychologists. I'd never been technically their
student, not on paper, though like Dr. Begum and Dr. Winkler they'd been nice enough to take me in, like wolves might
do for a human baby, bereft of its own species' elders.

It was the end, and the import of evaluations had fallen
away, and also a woman had died while waiting for admission to the psych ER, and everyone in Behavioral Health was
wrapped up in it—another in a line of travesties for an already
beleaguered staff. The Justice Department had been one thing,
and now this was a whole other. The psychiatrist on call in the
G Building ER in those early-morning hours had been fired
immediately: the security camera had recorded him "kicking"
the woman's still body, though I knew, we all did, that he was
only trying to safely rouse her. No matter that she had come
in and refused a medical exam (at least I'd overheard that),
it looked bad, and nothing was allowed to look bad without
people losing their jobs, a cynical and long-standing PR campaign that addressed nothing, until "nothing" was finally all

that ever got addressed. "At least it wasn't a resident on call," Dr. Singer said in hushed tones to Dr. Cherkesov from his seat in the CL conference room two buildings away.

It was late June, and we were leaving the hospital in a worse place than even when we got there, and us personally in this better place, so close to being done with all that school.

On my last day at CL, a week before the official final day as an intern at Kings County Hospital, I thanked Dr. Kapoor and Dr. Singer and Dr. Cherkesov for having me, for all that they had helped me to learn. Dr. Cherkesov asked how my time on CL had gone, and I told her it had been a lot to take in, just like the rest of internship. She nodded with her usual solemn face and then spoke in the voice that always matched it: "You will look back on your experience and discover so much more than you are able to grasp now."

CHAPTER ELEVEN

IT WAS THE END, AND EVERYTHING HAD TO BE COUNTED. How many patients we had seen and how many minutes we had spent with them and in what type of interaction. Psychologists are licensed by the state, and the best way the state could figure out to go about this was to quantify our training experiences, and to the minute. So I returned to CPEP in late June to look over the patient rosters from the month I'd spent there, hoping that I'd recall the names once I saw them so that I could copy them down to prove I'd put my time in. (Of course, we'd been advised at the beginning of the year to record the names and medical record numbers of all our patients, but things moved so quickly on most of the rotations, and none of us had done it. Now it was all over but the scrambling.)

I let myself into the psych ER with my skeleton key, and like moths to a flame my eyes rose to the familiar sign above its door: "If you don't have a key, you DON'T belong here." In

October, despite my key, I'd felt a certain kind of not belonging, one buttressed by my presumed shortcomings. Now I grasped the not belonging had origins also less particular to me, rooted in an institutional and ontological confusion and indifference. Both energized and worn down by this place that declared psychic problems medical ones and then sent me to go about some half-derided and under-supervised handling of them, I wouldn't hesitate to turn in the key, the last vestige of my official business there. But I would do it with a true ambivalence.

It was early, before 10:00, and the ER was quiet and bruised after the scrutiny it had come under following the death there. Post–Justice Department, the physical space looked altered, too. Doors were clearly marked: "Pediatric Suite," "Soiled Linens." It appeared cleaner and better lit, and there were fewer patients aimlessly milling about, though maybe June was just a quieter month. The place felt different now, and I felt different in it. The dread that had gathered in my stomach each time I'd arrived to spend my day inside back in the fall—so strongly I'd tried to overlook it—was gone now. I'd grown more comfortable behind locked doors, only now so close to when I would be rid of them. I went to the nursing station, where a closed-circuit television system had been installed and miniature TV screens let viewers see the goings-on of each remote corner of the place. I looked out from behind the thick glass and saw Mr. Rumbert, whom I'd first met in the psych ER and then followed to G-51. The immaculate pajamas I'd last seen him in on the unit had been replaced by plain jeans and a dark T-shirt. He looked upset, pacing and muttering and holding his arms tightly to his sides. At least he wasn't selectively mute. I walked out to greet him.

"Mr. Rumbert!" It was nice to see him but sad, too, as his very presence there could only mean things were not going well for him. He held still and looked at me.

"You ignored me before," he said. He sounded hurt. I hadn't seen him until just then, and I told him so. I tried to help calm him down, but after our initial greeting he just went back to his agitated pacing. The nurses on duty discussed giving him a sedative, less violent but slower acting than a shot. I hated to leave him like that, but I didn't work in the psych ER anymore, and anyway wasn't that always how it went?

I returned to my business. In a room in the back I'd rarely ventured into, I found a computer where old patient lists were saved as spreadsheets. I opened the documents dated each day I'd been there and scanned them. I'd been worried I wouldn't remember, but then I did and vividly, not only the names of the people I'd known eight months earlier and sometimes for just a day or two, but also even their stories. Angel Kingston, right, whose hallucinations started after a beating she got picking her kid up from school. Cyrus Varner, so sure that his neighbors were spies, with him their weaselly target. They'd impressed themselves upon me, these people, like footsteps on a beach. Time would eventually wash the particulars away, but it would have to be more than had already passed.

Time blurred other experiences more quickly, but maybe, too, that was willful on my part, like barely noticing the bodily dread engendered by the locked wards. When Scott conducted my end-of-year review, he emphasized how much better I'd gotten in the time since our last talk. I'd stopped railing against the scant attention paid to my training, and I'd been making an accompanying effort to look more cheerful besides (the latter with some resentment that this was what it took to be deemed a tolerable trainee). When I told the other interns about our meeting, they smiled and teased that finally I was reaping the rewards as opposed to the punishments of working under a boss with narcissistic tendencies: I was Scott's student, so after spending the year with him, I could only now be markedly improved. I laughed, too, but also felt kinder toward him than that. I imagined his words were his way of apologizing for whatever role he'd played in my difficulties there and of letting me know that he forgave my transgressions, too. In the end we were just two people growing uneasily into our roles.

That last morning there was a graduation party on the sixth floor, and all the psychologists came. Dr. Wolfe and Dr. Pine. Dr. T. and Dr. Levine. Dr. Winkler and Dr. Singer even dropped by, but not Dr. Begum, who had finally given up on getting G-51 into shape and fled to a child unit in J. The doctors talked to us like colleagues, I thought, though only Tamar would actually become that. She'd gotten the forensics job, the one I hadn't been interviewed for despite Dr. Wolfe's efforts ("What went on over there?" he'd asked me a month or so back, nodding his chin in the direction of Scott's office as I only shook my head). Scott and Dr. Reemer made speeches and gave us certificates of completion. Everyone applauded. The room had been decorated for the occasion, the streamers dangling from ceiling tiles only throwing into gross relief how unsuited for festivity the hard, rusted space actually was. I thought of the incoming intern class, who'd arrive to the streamers on Monday, full of envy for those of us who'd come—no, gone—before.

The interns would meet in Manhattan for celebratory drinks that night, but there was our individual business to be taken care of, and as always we went about that on our own. I finished late afternoon and knocked on Scott's door. I handed him my ID and my key, and we hugged because the moment required it, the embrace as necessary bookend. Caitlin came by and stood in the doorjamb, offering her own pale arms for a lukewarm pat. "Let us know what you're up to," she said as I moved down the hall.

The vestibule by the elevators was deserted. The sixth floor was Friday empty, and without any heavy metal to bang for the elevator, I hit its blue door with my house keys instead, producing a less than satisfying racket. There's something about leaving a place for the last time. I slowed down to take in the afternoon sunlight as it struggled through the dusky paned windows and hit the linoleum. I thought to remember the smell. When the elevator came, I got on. Two floors down a janitor boarded, and the operator showed him one of several Coach bags she'd stashed under her stool to sell. "Two hundred dollars," she said. "In the store they go for five hundred, but I get them stolen!" He bought it. There was a young lady he was trying to impress.

Outside on the street with a bursting feeling in my chest and nowhere in particular to be for a while, I was not sure what to do with myself and I called George. They were training him up to the last minute at his fancy private hospital, and my call went to voice mail.

"I'm done!" I cheered into the phone as I walked toward the subway that would spirit me away, but I didn't get the tone or the words quite right.

EPILOGUE

THERE IS VERY LITTLE DEMAND FOR NOT-YET-LICENSED PSY-chologists, and so I spent the summer after internship's end writing my dissertation, fact-checking at a soon-to-be-defunct magazine, and looking for a job, any job, in my field. (George had beaten me out for the one job we both interviewed for, screening applicants to the NYPD. I hated to lose any competition to my touched-by-the-Ivy-League husband, always so certain of the supremacy of his final training year, but at least I got health insurance out of the deal.) By October, I'd successfully defended and was ensconced at a public mental health clinic not far from home, being paid still very little to see outpatients by the dozen, putting in the hours I needed to fulfill my postdoctoral requirements for licensure.

It felt good doing long-term therapy again—what my training and interest best suited me for—and with people who usually wanted my services. The place was shabby but well run, with an attendance policy that made me think about Carmen Thompson and what kind of time we might have had together had Kings County's clinic maintained such a basic thing as that. (Maybe they'd expected too little from their charges, who then managed barely anything in return.) I did intake interviews as well as therapy at that clinic, and during those I realized this: no one who sat down across from me felt entirely unfamiliar. I could isolate, at least in broad strokes, what was going on with the most disturbed patients simply by sitting with them for a while and paying schooled attention, a not unnecessary skill for a clinical psychologist no matter the setting. In one of my few good moments with Caitlin Downs, around the middle of my internship year, she had said this, and it stuck with me: "At some point after you leave here, it will crystallize for you, what you got out of the experience." She'd been right and then some, as other lessons would become clearer as well, as time went by and I got around, learning again and again that graduate school had only been a very good beginning.

There were no such easy satisfactions for the G Building. Six months after I left, the Department of Justice issued its final report, which asserted that "significant and wide-ranging deficiencies exist with respect to Kings County Hospital's provision of care to its mental health patients." Among other things, it cited inadequate clinical leadership and under-staffing, "a system that has neither clear, specific standards of care nor an adequately trained supervisory, professional, and direct care staff." The hospital set out to hire a psychologist for each unit, though filling those positions proved difficult. G Building—a pointed threat for generations of neighbor-hood children—had a reputation.

The Justice Department made its suggestions, each quite reasonable on paper. Still, it was hard to imagine things getting better. Public hospitals are famously dysfunctional and stubborn places for dozens of social, political, and economic reasons well documented by others with much greater under-standing than mine. But there are also the psychological impediments to better treatment—at least as intractable and crossing socioeconomic lines. You can't call an orange an apple and then make a pie of it. Psychological problems are not simply medical ones (though I am hardly the first to observe this either). To mislabel the former the latter—in what has proved a failed attempt to obviate discomfort—results not in better treatment but its opposite. Ideally, we'd live in a world with less shame surrounding the sometimes-outsized travails of being human. Realistically, research will continue to con-firm that medication, even when it helps, is no stand-alone panacea, and the pendulum will swing back toward a wider valuing of the harder-won bounties psychologists offer.

After our year at Kings County Hospital, my fellow interns moved on to other things. Jen went to work with children in foster care. Alisa had a baby. Leora moved back to Israel. Zeke took a job in college counseling. Bruce left the field altogether, opening a beautiful mid-century modern furniture gallery on the East Side of Manhattan. Every few months Jen and I meet him there for dinner. We order Indian takeout, and talk eventually turns to the G Building, where in our wake Scott put Caitlin in charge of the externship program and then soon after got promoted himself.

Me, I would gladly work in a hospital again. In my fan-tasies, it's the hospital of my book, where interdisciplinary teams work together effectively, with respect for each other and a knowing certainty that patients who come for care will leave—as I did—having taken in some things worth knowing.

ACKNOWLEDGMENTS

With great appreciation for my dear sister, Cori Carr, who suggested I write this book, and then was also my perfect reader during the arduous process of writing it; and then, too, for Megan Abbott and Nana Asfour, for generosity with their thoughts, resources, and most of all friendship over many years. With gratitude to my parents, Michael and Helene Lockman, for many things, including their grace in the face of being undisguised subjects in their daughter's memoir. Thanks to Joe Reynoso, for going over this manuscript with a psychologist's eye. With love everlasting to my husband, George Kingsley, who, when this book began to feel like a quagmire, offered the best advice a nonfiction writer could get: "Write what happened." I feel incredibly lucky to have gotten the chance to work with both Dan Conaway—my agent and favorite cheerleader—and Gerry Howard, an editor whose wisdom always felt like that of a good therapist: ethereal, pragmatic, and exactly what I needed to hear at any given time. Finally, but not least, to my lovely fellow Kings County interns and the dozens of patients and professionals I had the opportunity to work with during my internship year. I was lucky to have known them all, even when that good fortune sometimes felt like something else along the way.